Long-Acting Injectable Medications in Mental Health

Megan J. Ehret

Long-Acting Injectable Medications in Mental Health

Springer

Megan J. Ehret
School of Pharmacy
University of Maryland
Baltimore, MD, USA

Editorial Contact: Jessica Chio

ISBN 978-3-032-09414-8 ISBN 978-3-032-09415-5 (eBook)
https://doi.org/10.1007/978-3-032-09415-5

This Springer imprint is published by the registered company Springer Nature Switzerland AG
The registered company address is: Gewerbestrasse 11, 6330 Cham, Switzerland

To those living with serious mental illness, whose strength and resilience in this world inspire me every step of this journey. May this work contribute to a future of greater understanding and extraordinary care.

To my husband, whose unwavering support, love, and belief in everything I do makes all things possible—this is for you, with endless gratitude.

To my children, whose joy, boundless energy, curiosity, and intellect remind me every day of the beauty in the world and the importance of hope. This is for you as well, with all my love.

And to my parents and family, you put me on this path and told me to "dream big." I hope I made your dreams come true—I still love you more than anything in the world.

Preface

Long-acting injectable (LAI) medications offer an important and often underutilized option in the treatment journey of many patients with mental health and substance use disorders. Their inclusion in our therapeutic toolbox opens new possibilities in managing chronic conditions such as schizophrenia, bipolar disorder, and substance use disorders, among other chronic illnesses.

I am often asked, "Which patients should receive an LAI?" or "Who would you recommend one for?" My answer is simple:

If I were newly diagnosed with osteoporosis, my provider would likely present me with treatment options—perhaps a daily pill, a weekly injection, or a periodic infusion. This conversation would happen without hesitation and without fear of how I might respond to the idea of an injectable or infusion-based treatment.

So why should we treat mental health or substance use disorders differently?

Every patient should be offered LAIs as a potential treatment—every time. Everyone is a candidate.

As healthcare providers, we are entrusted with guiding our patients toward the most appropriate treatment options for their unique needs. That includes treatments we may not be as familiar with or comfortable with. LAIs must be part of this conversation, always.

This book was written to support the entire interdisciplinary healthcare team. It aims to provide the tools and insights needed to confidently and effectively introduce LAIs into treatment plans. My hope is that it not only increases awareness and comfort with these formulations but also contributes to broader access and use of these valuable medications.

With greater understanding, we can expand access. And with expanded access, we can transform care.

This book offers a vital roadmap through the evolving landscape of long-acting injectables—empowering providers to shape the future of mental health and substance use disorder treatment.

Baltimore, MD, USA Megan J. Ehret

Competing Interests

Dr. Ehret has no competing interests to disclose.

Contents

About the Author

Megan J. Ehret is a graduate of the University of Toledo where she completed her BS and PharmD degrees, and she went on to complete a Psychiatric Pharmacy Residency at the Louis Stokes VAMC. She then completed a Psychopharmacology and Pharmacogenomics Fellowship at Nova Southeastern University. After training, she received her initial faculty appointment at the University of Connecticut and gained tenure during her stay there. While at the University of Connecticut, she served as the Vice-Chair of the IRB, Director of Practices for the Center for Correctional Health Networks, and a faculty member for the project: "ECHO: Buprenorphine." Currently, her full-time role is Professor, Vice-Chair of Academic Affairs, and Co-Director of the Mental Health Program at the University of Maryland School of Pharmacy with a practice site at The University of Maryland Mid Town Campus. Additionally, she also has the privilege of working with the State of Maryland Office of Pharmacy Services in evaluating antipsychotic use in the state, including development of clinical criteria for antipsychotics and authorizing and reviewing psychotropic use in the pediatric population. She is a Past-President of AAPP and is the current BCPP Recertification Director. She has worked with the State of Maryland to establish regulations permitting community pharmacists to administer maintenance injections. She has developed an interactive training program for students in administering long-acting injectable medications. She has numerous publications and book chapters describing psychotropic medication adherence and the role of pharmacogenomics in medication selection. Her current interests include psychotropic medication adherence and the advancement of psychiatric pharmacist practice.

Abbreviations

AUD	Alcohol Use Disorder
CrCl	Creatinine Clearance
IM	Intramuscular
LAI	Long-Acting Injectable
MOUD	Medications for Opioid Use Disorder
OUD	Opioid Use Disorder
REMS	Risk Evaluation and Mitigation Strategy
SAMHSA	Substance Abuse and Mental Health Services Administration
SQ	Subcutaneous
TMax	Time to Maximum Concentration

List of Figures

List of Tables

Chapter 1
Introduction to the Use of Long-Acting Injectable Antipsychotics

Introduction

Antipsychotic medications were developed in the 1950s, and poor adherence quickly became a critical concern for prescribers. The first long-acting injectable (LAI) antipsychotic medication, fluphenazine enanthate, was developed in 1966 due to the initiative of G. R. Daniels, with fluphenazine decanoate approximately 18 months later, to reduce the adverse effects from the enanthate formulation [1]. Haloperidol decanoate came to the market next in Europe in 1981 and in the United States in 1986 [2]. These medications demonstrated their benefit in the UK with the completion of two 'mirror image' studies, where the duration and frequency of admissions to the hospital were compared over identical periods before the use of LAIs and after the initial prescription. Although this design has many design flaws, it demonstrated a dramatic reduction in morbidity [3–5].

While novel in design, the concept of LAIs was not well received by medical professionals for fears of increased adverse effects, lack of efficacy, and the fear of imposition of treatment upon patients without regard to their feelings or rights [1]. Other psychiatrists didn't accept that LAIs would provide continuous coverage and thus provided oral overlap as a coverage strategy. However, the increasing concern regarding nonadherence in both those with serious mental illness and those with chronic illness motivated the gradual increase in the utilization of LAIs. Additionally, emerging scientific data has increased [6, 7, 8].

A series of double-blind prospective studies demonstrated the importance of LAIs in both chronic or relapsing schizophrenia and first-episode schizophrenia [9–20]. During a trial comparing oral and LAI fluphenazine, Hogarty et al. demonstrated that relapse rates were notably worse for patients taking the oral formulation, but this was not apparent until after at least a year of treatment [21]. This led to the growth of outpatient use of LAIs worldwide [22]. The use varied in different countries, with the highest use in the UK, followed by Sweden and Austria [23–25].

M. J. Ehret, *Long-Acting Injectable Medications in Mental Health*,
https://doi.org/10.1007/978-3-032-09415-5_1

Germany and the United States had the lowest use, likely due to delivery problems, with reliance on general practitioners and other professionals to administer the medications.

Consequences of Nonadherence to Antipsychotic Treatment and Current Treatment Guidelines

While the definition of medication adherence is variable, recent definitions have suggested that ≥80% of medication taken over 12 months and/or <1 week missed medication (over 3 months) [26]. Studies have demonstrated that nonadherence rates to oral medications in patients with schizophrenia are as high as 50% [27]. Additionally, adherence behavior fluctuates over time during schizophrenia and should be considered a core aspect of the illness [28]. Poor medication adherence is a risk factor for relapses in both chronic and first-episode illness [29, 30]. Most hospital readmissions for those with schizophrenia typically have some degree of nonadherence associated with them [31]. Improvements in clinical symptoms and functioning, a reduction in the use of concomitant medications, the rate of hospitalization, and the duration of hospital stay, have been correlated with better adherence [32]. Patients who are adherent have also demonstrated significantly lower hospital costs [33, 34].

The first guidelines for the treatment of schizophrenia recommended that LAIs should be considered for "any patients with schizophrenia for whom long-term treatment is indicated." [35] Several other sets of guidelines only recommended LAIs for patients with recurrent relapses related to partial or full nonadherence, or in patients with persistent positive symptoms [36, 37]. Over time, evidence has shifted, and recommendations suggest that LAIs should not be restricted to just patients with adherence problems but instead should be offered more widely through shared decision-making strategies [38, 39]. The current American Psychiatric Association Schizophrenia treatment guidelines recommend LAIs for those patients who demonstrate nonadherence to oral medications or those who prefer the medication formulation [40].

Advantages and Disadvantages of LAIs

There are many potential advantages to the use of LAIs in the treatment of schizophrenia [41–45]:

- Reduction in dosage deviations over the course of treatment
- Potential elimination of questionable adherence status
- Decreased need for the patient to take daily oral medication(s)
- Establishment of the date of nonadherence should an injection appointment be missed

- Disentanglement for the rationale of poor response due to nonadherence
- Establishment of a relationship between the dose and therapeutic drug monitoring
- Predicted plasma levels
- Potential elimination of abrupt loss of efficacy if an injection is missed
- Decreasing hospitalizations
- Preventing relapses
- Decreasing mortality

While there are many advantages to the use of LAIs, some disadvantages have been identified in the literature, including the following [45–49]:

- Slower dose titrations
- Longer time to achieve steady state levels
- Less flexibility of dose adjustments
- Delayed disappearance of distressing and/or severe adverse effects
- Pain at the injection site can occur, and leakage into the subcutaneous tissue and/or the skin may cause irritation and lesions
- Burden of frequent travel to outpatient clinics or home visits by community nurses for their administration
- May require refrigeration and/or reconstitution
- Perception of stigma

Many of these identified disadvantages have been addressed with newer formulations of LAIs, including loading dose strategies, flexibility of dosing adjustments, increased clinic access, and less stigma at injection sites.

When weighing the risks and benefits of using an LAI, providers should be aware that patients are willing to accept an LAI when they are properly informed regarding the benefits of the formulation. In a survey of psychiatrists, patient refusal was cited as a primary reason for not prescribing LAIs [50]. However, in a survey of patients without LAI experience, 79% cited having never been informed about the option by their psychiatrist, and 75% of psychiatrists felt that they informed the patient, but only 33% of patients felt informed [51]. Moreover, in a survey of patients with greater than 3 months of LAI experience, injectable medications were the preferred formulation, and 70% of patients felt better supported in their illness by virtue of regular contact with the doctor or nurse who administered their injection [52].

Considerations for When to Select an LAI

When considering the use of an LAI for a patient, there are several factors to consider:

- Is the patient demonstrating adequate efficacy and tolerability on oral fluphenazine, haloperidol, risperidone, paliperidone, olanzapine, or aripiprazole?

- With appropriate discussion and shared decision-making, the provider should offer and switch the patient to the corresponding LAI formulation.
- Engaging the patient in discussions with questions such as: "How would you like to take your medication once a month?" should be undertaken.

- Is the patient being treated acutely?
  - Consider an LAI that does not require oral supplementation.
- What adverse effects are of concern for this individual patient (e.g., metabolic syndrome or movement disorders)?
- Are prolactin-related adverse effects a clinical concern for this individual patient? Consider avoiding risperidone-based products.
- Is acquisition cost the primary concern? Consider using a generic product [53].

Other items to consider when selecting an LAI include who will administer the medication, what dose will be required, what will the injection volume be and whether the patient can tolerate the injection, what site will be utilized for the injection, whether the patient has concerns regarding the potential need for oral overlap when initiating the medication, and what the medication storage requirements are for the injection. Additionally, the provider should consider the recommendations for re-initiation in the event that the patient misses an injection.

How to Approach the Discussion of LAIs with Patients

Offering an LAI medication requires a thoughtful and informative approach that prioritizes shared decision-making and trauma-informed care. It is crucial to present the formulation as a beneficial option, and not as a last resort or punishment for nonadherence. Providers should be aware of any trauma history a patient may have, as this can be a factor in why a patient may not choose an injectable medication. Establishing a therapeutic relationship should occur when the provider is able to initiate the conversation regarding an LAI medication. Providers should introduce the LAI early in the disease process. Anyone with a new diagnosis, recent relapse, or who is transitioning from inpatient care or incarceration should be offered an LAI. The conversation should focus on the benefits of the LAIs and why they may be a good fit for the patient. These can include discussions regarding improving adherence, reducing relapse and hospitalization, maintaining steady medication levels, and improving the quality of life of the patient. Providers should convey a clear, optimistic message regarding the formulation. The opportunity should be provided to the patient to ask questions, and the provider should address any misconceptions the patient may have. When involving the patient in the shared decision-making process, the provider is offering an LAI as an alternative to other treatment options, discussing the pros and cons of each option. The provider should consider the individual preferences of the patient, including the injection site and interval length for injections. Working together to collaborate on a plan permits the patient and provider to align their goals and strategies for treatment.

After the agreement, the provider should provide the patient with practical information regarding the injection process, including how the injection is administered, the site of injection, and the frequency of injection. The initiation protocols should be reviewed, and if oral supplementation is required, the duration should be determined. The potential adverse effects and mitigation strategies should be reviewed. Additionally, cost and insurance coverage should be verified. Patients should also be informed about any necessary postinjection monitoring and follow-up appointments [54].

Conclusion

In patients with schizophrenia, preventing relapse is critically important, as it is associated with progressive frontal gray matter loss, increased hospital readmissions, higher suicide rates, and rising healthcare costs. Early and sustained prevention can significantly impact a patient's long-term outcomes. Adherence to antipsychotic treatment plays a key role in reducing relapse risk, making it essential for providers to identify and address barriers to adherence. LAIs have been shown to lower the risk of relapse and hospitalization, and a growing number of LAI options are now available. Individuals in the early stages of illness stand to benefit the most—and have the most to lose—highlighting the importance of this timely intervention.

References

1. Johnson D. Historical perspective on antipsychotic long-acting injections. Br J Psychiatry. 2009;195:S7–S12.
2. Knudsen P. Chemotherapy with neuroleptics: clinical and pharmacokinetic aspects with a particular view to depot preparations. Acta Psychiatr Scand. 1985;72(Suppl 322):51–7.
3. Denham J, Adamson L. The contribution of fluphenazine enanthate and decanoate in the prevention of readmission of schizophrenic patients. Acta Psychiatr Scand. 1971;47:420–30.
4. Johsnon DAW, Freeman HL. Long-acting tranquillisers. Practitioner. 1972;208:395–400.
5. Gottfries GC, Green L. Fluphenthixol decanoate- in treatment of out-patients. Acta Psychiatr Scand Suppl. 1974;225:15–24.
6. Hogarty GE, Goldberg SC, Schooler NR. Drug and sociotherapy in the aftercare of schizophrenic patients: one year relapse rates. Arch Gen Psychiatry. 1973;28:54–64.
7. Hogarty GE, Goldberg SC, Schooler NR. Drug and sociotherapy in the aftercare of schizophrenic patients: two year relapse rates. Arch Gen Psychiatry. 1974;31:603–8.
8. Hogarty GE, Ulrich R, Goldberg SC. Sociotherapy and the prevention of relapse among schizophrenic patients. In: Spitzer RL, Klein DF, editors. Evaluation of psychological therapies. Baltimore: Johns Hopkins Press; 1976. p. 283–93.
9. Hirsch SR, Gaind R, Rhode PD, et al. Outpatient maintenance of chronic schizophrenic patients with long acting phenothiazines. BMJ. 1973;i:633–7.

10. Davis JM. Overview: maintenance therapy in schizophrenia. I. Schizophrenia. Am J Psychiatry. 1975;132:1237–45.
11. Rifkin A, Quitkin F, Rabiner CJ. Fluphenazine decanoate, fluphenazine hydrochloride given orally and placebo in remitted schizophrenia: relapse rate over one year. Arch Gen Psychiatry. 1977;34:43–7.
12. Quitkin F, Rifkin A, Kane J, et al. Long-acting oral drugs vs. injectable antipsychotic drugs in schizophrenia: a one year double-blind comparison in multi episode schizophrenia. Arch Gen Psychiatry. 1978;35:889–92.
13. Schooler NR, Levine J, Severe JB, et al. Prevention of relapse in schizophrenia: an evaluation of fluphenzaine decanoate. Arch Gen Psychiatry. 1980;37:16–24.
14. Tegeler J, Lehmann E. A follow-up study of schizophrenic outpatients treated with depot neuroleptics. Prog Neuropsycopharmacol. 1981;5:79–90.
15. Wistedt B. A neuroleptic withdrawal study in chronic schizophrenic patients. Acta Psychiatr Scand. 1981;64:65–84.
16. Kane JM, Rifkin A, Quitkin F, et al. Fluphenazine versus placebo in patients with remitted, acute first episodes of schizophrenia. Arch Gen Psychaitry. 1982;39:70–3.
17. Johnson DAW. Depression: treatment compliance in general practice. Acta Psychiatr Scand Suppl. 1983;63(Suppl 290):447–53.
18. Johnson DAW. Observations on the use of long-acting depot neuroleptic injections in the maintenance treatment of schizophrenia. J Clin Psychiatry. 1984;45:13–21.
19. Crow TJ, McMillan JF, Johnson AL, et al. A randomized controlled trial of prophylactic neuroleptic treatment. Br J Psychiatry. 1986;148:120–7.
20. Pietzcker A, Gaebel W, Kopcke W, et al. A German multicenter study on the neuroleptic long-term therapy of schizophrenic patients. Pharmacopsychiatry. 1986;19:161–6.
21. Hogarty GE, Scholler NR, Ulrich R, et al. Fluphenazine and social therapy in the aftercare of schizophrenic patients. Relapse analyses of a two-year controlled study of fluphenazine decanoate and fluphenazine hydrochloride. Arch Gen Psychiatry. 1979;36:1283–94.
22. Kissling W. Neuroleptic relapse prevention. In: Guidelines for neuroleptic relapse prevention in schizophrenia. Heidelberg: Springer; 1991. p. 50–2.
23. Johnson DAW. United Kingdom: neuroleptic relapse prevention. In: Kissling W, editor. Guidelines for neuroleptic relapse prevention in schizophrenia. Heidelberg: Springer; 1991. p. 45.
24. Dencker SJ. Sweden: neuroleptic relapse prevention. In: Kissling W, editor. Guidelines for neuroleptic relapse prevention in schizophrenia. Heidelberg: Springer; 1991. p. 24.
25. Fleischhacker WW, Meise U. Austria: the current state of maintenance treatment of schizophrenia. In: Kissling W, editor. Guidelines for neuroleptic relapse prevention in schizophrenia. Heidelberg: Springer; 1991. p. 13.
26. Velligan DI, Diamond P, Mueller J, et al. The short-term impact of generic versus individualized environmental supports on functional outcomes and target behaviors in schizophrenia. Psychiatry Res. 2009;168:94–101.
27. Glazer WM, Byerly MJ. Tactics and technologies to manage nonadherence in patients with schizophrenia. Curr Psychiatry Rep. 2008;20:359–69.
28. Weiden PJ. Understanding and addressing adherence issues in schizophrenia: from theory to practice. J Clin Psychiatry. 2007;68:14–9.
29. Valenstein M, Copeland LA, Blow FC, et al. Pharmacy data identify poorly adherent patients with schizophrenia at increased risk for admission. Med Care. 2002;40:630–9.
30. Morkin G, Widen JH, Grawe RW. Non-adherence to antipsychotic medication, relapse and rehospitalization in recent-onset schizophrenia. BMC Psychiatry. 2008;8:32.
31. Kane JM, Garcia-Ribera C. Clinical guideline recommendations for antipsychotic long-acting injections. Br J Psychiatry Suppl. 2009;52:S63–7.
32. Olivares JM, Peuskens J, Pecanak J, et al. Clinical and resource-use outcomes of risperidone long-acting injection in recent and long-term diagnosed schizophrenia patients: results from a multinational electronic registry. Curr Med Res Opin. 2009;25:2197–206.

33. Gilmer TP, Dolder CR, Lacro JP, et al. Adherence to treatment with antipsychotic medication and health care costs among Medicaid beneficiaries with schizophrenia. Am J Psychiatry. 2004;161:692–9.
34. Dilla T, Ciudad A, Alvarez M. Systematic review of the economic aspects of nonadherence to antipsychotic medication in patients with schizophrenia. Patient Prefer Adherence. 2013;4:275–84.
35. Kane JM, Aguglia E, Altamura AC, et al. Guidelines for depot antipsychotic treatment in schizophrenia. European Neuropsychopharmacology consensus conference in Siena, Italy. Eur Neuropsychopharmacol. 1998;8:55–66.
36. Lehman AF, Lieberman JA, Dixon LB, et al. Practice guideline for the treatment of patients with schizophrenia, second edition. Am J Psychiatry. 2004;161:1–56.
37. Canadian Psychiatric Association. Clinical practice guidelines. Treatment of schizophrenia. Can J Psychiatr. 2005;50:7S–57S.
38. Uribe ES, Mundo SEO, Garza RRM, et al. Comparative safety of long-acting injectable antipsychotics: a systematic review and network meta-analysis. Psychiatry Investig. 2023;20:1112–25.
39. Llorca PM, Abbar M, Courtet P, et al. Guidelines for the use and management of long-acting injectable antipsychotics in serious mental illness. BMC Psychiatry. 2013;20:340.
40. Keepers GA, Fochtmann LJ, Anzia JM, et al. The American Psychiatric Association Practice Guideline for the treatment of patients with schizophrenia. Am J Psychiatry. 2020;77:868–72.
41. McEvoy JP. Risks and benefits of different types of long-acting injectable antipsychotics. J Clin Psychiatry. 2006;67:15–8.
42. Olfson M, Marcus SC, Ascher-Svanum H. Treatment of schizophrenia with long-acting fluphenazine, haloperidol, or risperidone. Schizophr Bull. 2007;33:1379–87.
43. Kane JM. Strategies for improving compliance in treatment of schizophrenia by using a long-acting formulation of an antipsychotic: clinical studies. J Clin Psychiatry. 2003;64:34–40.
44. Patel MX, DE Zoysa N, Baker D, et al. Antipsychotic depot medication and attitudes of community psychiatric nurses. J Psychiatr Ment Health Nurs. 2005;12:237–44.
45. Heres S, Schmitz FS, Leucht S, et al. The attitude of patients towards antipsychotic depot treatment. Int Clin Psychopharmacol. 2007;22:275–85.
46. Remington GJ, Adams ME. Depot neuroleptic therapy: clinical considerations. Can J Psychiatr. 1995;40:S5–11.
47. Knox ED, Stimmel GL. Clinical review of a long-acting, injectable formulation of risperidone. Clin Ther. 2004;26:1994–2002.
48. Gerlach J. Depot neuroleptics in relapse prevention: advantages and disadvantages. Int Clin Psychopharmacol. 1995;5:17–20.
49. Brissos S, Veguilla MR, Taylor D, et al. The role of long-acting injectable antipsychotics in schizophrenia: a critical appraisal. Ther Adv Psychopharmacol. 2014;4:198–219.
50. Heres S, Hamann J, Kissling W, et al. Attitudes of psychiatrists toward antipsychotic depot medication. J Clin Psychiatry. 2006;67:1948–53.
51. Jaeger M, Rossler W. Attitudes towards long-acting depot antipsychotics: a survey of patients, relatives and psychiatrists. Psychiatry Res. 2010;175:58–62.
52. Caroli F, Raymondet P, Izard I, et al. Opinions of French patients with schizophrenia regarding injectable medications. Patient Prefer Adherence. 2011;21:165–71.
53. Citrome L. New second-generation long-acting injectable antipsychotics for the treatment of schizophrenia. Expert Rev Neurother. 2013;13:767–83.
54. Guide to long-acting medications. National Council for Mental Wellbeing; 2025.

Chapter 2
Fluphenazine Decanoate: First-Generation Antipsychotic Long-Acting Injectable

LAI Technology

Fluphenazine decanoate consists of an ester of the active medication held in a sesame seed oil suspension [1, 2]. The antipsychotic medication, fluphenazine, is combined with a long-chain fatty acid in a process called esterification. This process makes fluphenazine soluble, so it can be dissolved in the sesame seed oil. Once injected intramuscularly, the medication slowly leaves the oil reservoir, and in the bloodstream, the antipsychotic is separated from the fatty acid [3].

Per the package insert labeling, fluphenazine decanoate injection is a long-acting parenteral antipsychotic Food and Drug Administration (FDA)-approved for use in the management of patients requiring prolonged parenteral neuroleptic therapy (e.g., chronic schizophrenia). Fluphenazine decanoate injection has not been shown to be effective in the management of behavioral complications in patients with mental retardation [3].

Dosing Parameters

As with all long-acting injectables (LAIs), establishment of tolerability with prior oral administration is recommended prior to utilization of the LAI formulation. Table 2.1 provides the dosing recommendations for fluphenazine decanoate.

Fluphenazine decanoate has an established conversion of the oral formulation to the LAI formulation. Table 2.2 provides the dose conversion of oral fluphenazine to fluphenazine decanoate [3].

If an individual should miss a scheduled injection of fluphenazine decanoate, an established missed dose schedule is not provided by the package labeling. Based on pharmacokinetic parameters of the medication, clinical recommendations are

M. J. Ehret, *Long-Acting Injectable Medications in Mental Health*,
https://doi.org/10.1007/978-3-032-09415-5_2

Table 2.1 Dosing recommendations [3]

Initial dose	12.5–25 mg IM/SQ
Oral overlap	Continue oral, decreasing dose by half after first injection, discontinue oral therapy after second injection
Target dose	12.5–50 mg every 2–4 weeks (interval determined by patient response)
Maximum dose	100 mg every 2 weeks
Dosing interval	Every 2–4 weeks
Renal/hepatic dosing	None noted in package insert

IM intramuscular, *SQ* subcutaneous

Table 2.2 Dose conversion of oral to decanoate

Oral dose	LAI dose
10 mg	12.5 decanoate every 3 weeks

LAI long-acting injectable antipsychotic medication

Table 2.3 Missed dose recommendations [4]

Time from last dose	How to manage
Patient at steady state and ≤6 weeks from last dose	Administer the next dose as soon as possible
Patient not at steady state, or it has been >6 to 24 weeks since last dose	Plasma levels may fall lower than the therapeutic window Give the next injection as soon as possible Provide oral antipsychotic medication supplementation if there is symptom recurrence Within the first 24 h after injection (time to peak), monitor for adverse effects
>24 weeks since the last injection	Stabilize on an oral antipsychotic medication Fluphenazine decanoate should be reinitiated

available for consideration on how to manage this situation. Table 2.3 provides clinical recommendations on how to manage missed doses of fluphenazine decanoate.

Pharmacokinetic Properties

Fluphenazine decanoate levels peak 24 h after the injection [5]. A study evaluating fluphenazine decanoate levels after discontinuation of the LAI found no significant difference in plasma levels 6 weeks after the last dose of fluphenazine decanoate, but a significant decrease in levels was found at 8–12 weeks after the last dose [6]. Additional studies have found that fluphenazine levels are still detectable from 21 to 24 weeks following discontinuation of the LAI [7, 8]. Plasma concentrations do not decline smoothly, likely due to "lumps" in residual release from previous injection sites or multicompartment redistribution.

Table 2.4 Pharmacokinetic properties [3, 9]

Half-life	Single injection of 25 mg: 6.8–9.6 days Multiple injections: 14.3 days ± 2.2 days
TMax	2–4 days
Time to steady state	4–6 weeks
Therapeutic window	0.2–2 ng/mL

TMax time to maximum concentration

There may be a significant amount of fluphenazine decanoate released early or "dose dumping," which may result in high peak plasma concentrations that occur within the first day of injection. Close monitoring of adverse effects should be done after the first injection. Pharmacokinetic properties of fluphenazine decanoate are provided in Table 2.4.

Drug Interactions

Fluphenazine decanoate may be affected by CYP2D6 metabolizer status, but no dose adjustment information is available in the package insert [3].

Adverse Effects

Fluphenazine decanoate has similar adverse effects to other first-generation antipsychotic medications [10, 11]. Common adverse effects include sedation, dry mouth, dry eyes, blurred vision, constipation, orthostasis, dizziness, hypotension, and urinary retention. Due to the dopaminergic antagonism mechanism of action, fluphenazine can cause extrapyramidal symptoms and tardive dyskinesia [12].

Preparation and Administration Instructions

The decanoate is available in a 25 mg/mL strength 5 mL multidose vial in a sesame oil vehicle with 12 mg benzyl alcohol as a preservative [3]. Syringes and needles are not provided with the vial, so the provider must obtain those prior to administration. Needles of 21-gauge or larger are recommended.

This decanoate doesn't require any reconstitution or refrigeration. The vial should be stored with protection from light.

Injection site: Gluteal or deltoid muscle

Injection volume: This is dependent on the dose. Doses larger than 3 mL per injection site should not be administered.

Administration instructions:

- As a universal precaution, hands should be washed with soap and water. Gloves should always be worn.
- Verification that the patient doesn't have an allergy to sesame seeds should occur. The vial should be visually inspected for particulate matter and discoloration prior to administration, whenever the solution and container permit.
- Due to the sesame seed oil vehicle, the solution should be pulled out of the vial with a larger gauge needle (i.e., 18 gauge) and then injected with a new, smaller gauge needle (i.e., 21 gauge) for the patient's comfort.
- The Z-track administration technique is recommended [13].
  - The Z-track method prevents the oil medication from leaking out of the muscle and into the subcutaneous tissue after the injection.
  - Additionally, this method can reduce pain and irritation at the injection site.
  - With the nondominant hand, pull the skin and subcutaneous tissue laterally (away from the injection site) about 1–1.5 inches.
  - Using the dominant hand, insert the needle into the muscle at a 90° angle.
  - Slowly inject the medication as prescribed.
  - Quickly withdraw the needle at the same angle it was inserted.
  - Immediately release the skin and tissue, allowing the displaced tissue to slide back into place.
  - Apply gentle pressure to the injection site with a gauze pad.
- Postinjection monitoring should include blood pressure due to the risk of hypotension.
- Dispose of the syringe in an appropriate sharps container.

References

1. Marder SR, Putten T, Aravagiri M, et al. Fluphenazine plasma levels and clinical response. Psychopharmacol Bull. 1990;26:256–9.
2. Kurland AA, Richardson JH. A comparative study of two long acting phenothiazine preparations, fluphenazine enanthate and fluphenazine decanoate. Psychopharmacologia (Berl). 1966;9:320–7.
3. Fluphenazine Decanoate Injection. USP [package insert]. Rockford: Mylan Institutional LLC; 2018.
4. Carpenter J, Wong KK. Use a stepwise approach based on the unique properties of the specific medication. Curr Psychiatr Ther. 2018;17:11–20.
5. Ereshefsky L, Saklad SR, Jann MW. Future of depot neuroleptic therapy: pharmacokinetic and pharmacodynamic approaches. J Clin Psychiatry. 1984;45:50–8.
6. Gitlin MJ, Midha KK, Fogelson D, et al. Persistence of fluphenazine in plasma after decanoate withdrawal. J Clin Psychopharmacol. 1988;8:53–6.
7. Wistedt B, Wiles D, Kolakowska T. Slow decline of plasma drug and prolactin levels after discontinuation of chronic treatment with depot neuroleptics. Lancet. 1981;1:1163.
8. Wistedt B, Jorgensen A, Wiles D. A depot neuroleptic withdrawal study. Plasma concentration of fluphenazine and flupenthixol and relapse frequency. Psychopharmacology. 1982;78:301–4.

9. Jann MW, Ereshefsky L, Saklad SR. Clinical pharmacokinetics of the depot antipsychotics. Clin Pharmacokinet. 1985;10:315–33.
10. Knights A, Okasha MS, Salih MA, et al. Depressive and extrapyramidal symptoms and clinical effects: a trial of fluphenazine versus fluphenthixol in maintenance of schizophrenic outpatients. Br J Psychiatry. 1979;135:515–23.
11. Alarcon R, Carney MWP. Severe depressive mood changes following slow-release intramuscular fluphenazine injection. Br Med J. 1969;3:564–7.
12. Maayan N, Quaraishi SN, David A, et al. Fluphenazine decanoate (depot) and enanthate for schizophrenia. Cochrane Database Syst Rev. 2015;5:CD000307.
13. Pullen RL. Administering medication by Z-track method. Nursing. 2005;35:24.

Chapter 3
Haloperidol Decanoate: First-Generation Antipsychotic Long-Acting Injectable

LAI Technology

Haloperidol decanoate consists of an ester of the active medication held in a sesame seed oil suspension. The antipsychotic medication, haloperidol, is combined with a long-chain fatty acid in a process called esterification. This process makes haloperidol soluble, so it is able to be dissolved in sesame seed oil. Once injected intramuscularly, the medication slowly leaves the oil reservoir, and in the bloodstream, the antipsychotic is separated from the fatty acid [1].

Per the package insert labeling, haloperidol decanoate is indicated for the treatment of patients with schizophrenia who require prolonged parenteral antipsychotic therapy [1].

Dosing Parameters

As with all long-acting injectable (LAIs), establishment of tolerability with prior oral administration is recommended prior to utilization of the LAI formulation. Table 3.1 provides the dosing recommendations for haloperidol decanoate.

Haloperidol decanoate has an established conversion of the oral formulation to the LAI formulation. Table 3.2 provides the dose conversion of oral haloperidol to haloperidol decanoate.

If an individual should miss a scheduled injection of haloperidol decanoate, an established missed dose schedule is not provided by the package labeling. Based on pharmacokinetic parameters of the medication, clinical recommendations are available for consideration on how to manage this situation. Table 3.3 provides clinical recommendations on how to manage missed doses of haloperidol decanoate.

M. J. Ehret, *Long-Acting Injectable Medications in Mental Health*,
https://doi.org/10.1007/978-3-032-09415-5_3

Table 3.1 Dosing recommendations [1, 2]

Initial dose	Conventional dose: 10–15 times the current oral daily dose Loading dose: 20 times the current oral daily dose (recommended for those on an oral dose >10 mg/day, who have a risk of relapses or who have long-term use resulting in tolerance), the initial dose should be reduced in the second month to avoid accumulation Second loading dose strategy: Load with weekly injections over 1 month with no oral coverage except for the first week. Conversion formulation is 10 mg/day = weekly injections of 100 mg. The maintenance dose would be 20 times the current oral dose and would be given 2 weeks after the last loading injection. If injection dose conversion is >100 mg, a second injection should be administered in 3–7 days. The second dose would be the loading dose minus the first dose given.
Oral overlap	Continue the oral dose for the first two to three injections if not using a loading dose
Target dose	10–15 times daily oral dose IM every 4 weeks
Maximum dose	100 mg/first injection; 450 mg/4 weeks based on limited clinical experience at greater doses
Dosing interval	Every 4 weeks; If the maintenance dose exceeds 300 mg, then divide the dose and administer every 14 days.
Renal/hepatic dosing	None noted in package insert

IM intramuscular

Table 3.2 Dose conversion of oral to decanoate [1]

Conventional dose: LAI is 10–15 times the current oral daily dose

LAI long-acting injectable antipsychotic medication

Table 3.3 Missed dose recommendations [3]

Time from last dose	How to manage
Patient at steady state and ≤6 weeks since the last injection	Administer the next injection as soon as possible
Patient not at steady state, or it has been >6 to 12 weeks since last dose	Plasma levels may fall lower than the therapeutic window Give the next injection as soon as possible Provide oral antipsychotic medication supplementation if there is symptom recurrence Around Day 6, after injection (time to peak), monitor for adverse effects
≥13 weeks since the last injection	Stabilize on an oral antipsychotic medication Haloperidol decanoate should be reinitiated

Table 3.4 Pharmacokinetic properties

Half-life	8–14 days
TMax	3–9 days
Time to steady state	3–4 months
Therapeutic window	3–15 ng/mL

TMax time to maximum concentration

Pharmacokinetic Properties

Haloperidol decanoate plasma concentrations typically peak on the seventh day following injection, but may peak on the first day. The reduced metabolite of haloperidol is present in significant quantities in those receiving the oral preparation, but this has not been reported in the pharmacokinetic studies with the depot preparation. While the therapeutic range has been reported to be 3–40 ng/mL in several studies, these studies did not measure the reduced metabolite. It has been proposed that the presence of high concentrations of the reduced metabolite may affect the response to haloperidol. Pharmacokinetic properties of haloperidol decanoate are provided in Table 3.4 [1, 4].

Drug Interactions

Haloperidol decanoate may be mildly to moderately increased when given concomitantly with medications characterized as substrates or inhibitors of CYP3A4 or CYP2D6 isoenzymes [1].

Adverse Effects

Specific adverse reactions from haloperidol decanoate are the same as those of other dosage forms of haloperidol, which are similar to other first-generation antipsychotic medications. Common adverse effects include sedation, dry mouth, dry eyes, blurred vision, constipation, orthostasis, dizziness, hypotension, and urinary retention. Due to the dopaminergic antagonism mechanism of action, haloperidol can cause extrapyramidal symptoms and tardive dyskinesia [4].

Preparation and Administration Instructions

The decanoate is available in 50 mg/mL and 100 mg/mL strengths in 1 mL single-dose vials and 5 mL multidose vials in sesame oil vehicle with 1.2% benzyl alcohol as a preservative. Syringes and needles are not provided with the vial, so the provider must obtain them prior to administration. Needles of 21-gauge or larger are recommended [1].

This decanoate doesn't require any reconstitution or refrigeration. The vial should be stored with protection from light.

Injection site: Gluteal or deltoid muscle

Injection volume: This is dependent on the dose. Doses larger than 3 mL per injection site should not be administered.

Administration instructions:

- As a universal precaution, hands should be washed with soap and water. Gloves should always be worn.
- Verification that the patient doesn't have an allergy to sesame seeds should occur. The vial should be visually inspected for particulate matter and discoloration prior to administration, whenever the solution and container permit.
- Verification of the strength ordered and the vial selected prior to administration to verify that the correct dose is given. This step is completed to verify that an appropriate volume is administered (i.e., 50 mg/mL for a 400 mg injection would result in an 8 mL injection, versus a 100 mg/mL for a 400 mg injection would result in a 4 mL injection)
- Due to the sesame seed oil vehicle, the solution should be pulled out of the vial with a larger gauge needle (i.e., 18 gauge) and then injected with a new, smaller gauge (i.e., 21 gauge) for the patient's comfort.
- The Z-track administration technique is recommended [5].
  - The Z-track method prevents the oil medication from leaking out of the muscle and into the subcutaneous tissue after the injection.
  - Additionally, this method can reduce pain and irritation at the injection site.
  - With the nondominant hand, pull the skin and subcutaneous tissue laterally (away from the injection site) about 1–1.5 inches.
  - Using the dominant hand, insert the needle into the muscle at a 90° angle.
  - Slowly inject the medication as prescribed.
  - Quickly withdraw the needle at the same angle it was inserted.
  - Immediately release the skin and tissue, allowing the displaced tissue to slide back into place.
  - Apply gentle pressure to the injection site with a gauze pad.
- Postinjection monitoring should include blood pressure due to the risk of hypotension.
- Dispose of the syringe in an appropriate sharps container.

References

1. Haloperidol decanoate injection [package insert]. North Wales: TEVA Pharmaceuticals; 2019.
2. Meyer JM. A rational approach to employing high plasma levels of antipsychotics for violence associated with schizophrenia: case vignettes. CNS Spectr. 2014;19:422–38.

3. Carpenter J, Wong KK. Use a stepwise approach based on the unique properties of the specific medication. Curr Psychiatr Ther. 2018;17:11–20.
4. Hemstrom CA, Evans RL, Lobeck FG. Haloperidol decanoate: a depot antipsychotic. Drug Intell Clin Pharm. 1988;22:290–5.
5. Pullen RL. Administering medication by Z-track method. Nursing. 2005;35:24.

Chapter 4
Aripiprazole Monohydrate (Abilify Maintena®): Second-Generation Antipsychotic Long-Acting Injectable

LAI Technology

Abilify Maintena® is a lyophilized powder of unmodified aripiprazole, which is constituted in sterile water to an aqueous suspension. Due to the low solubility of the aripiprazole particles, following intramuscular (IM) injection, aripiprazole is absorbed into the systemic circulation slowly [1].

Per the package insert labeling, Abilify Maintena® is an atypical antipsychotic indicated for the treatment of schizophrenia in adults and for maintenance monotherapy treatment of bipolar I disorder in adults [1].

Dosing Parameters

As with all long-acting injectable (LAIs), establishment of tolerability with prior oral administration is recommended prior to utilization of the LAI formulation. It has been noted that it may take up to 14 days to complete the tolerability testing due to the long half-life of aripiprazole (i.e., 75 h and 94 h for aripiprazole and dehydro-aripiprazole, respectively). Table 4.1 provides dosing recommendations for Abilify Maintena® [1].

Abilify Maintena® has an established conversion of the oral formulation to the LAI formulation. Table 4.2 provides the dose conversion of oral aripiprazole to Abilify Maintena® [1, 2].

If an individual misses a scheduled injection of Abilify Maintena®, an established missed dose schedule has been established within the package labeling. Table 4.3 provides clinical recommendations on how to manage missed doses of Abilify Maintena®.

M. J. Ehret, *Long-Acting Injectable Medications in Mental Health*, https://doi.org/10.1007/978-3-032-09415-5_4

Table 4.1 Dosing recommendations [1]

Initial dose	1-day initiation: Administer 2 IM injections of Abilify Maintena® 400 mg in two different injection sites (in either the deltoid or gluteal muscle), and one dose of oral aripiprazole 20 mg on the first day of treatment with Abilify Maintena® 14-day initiation: When Abilify Maintena® is initiated in patients receiving oral aripiprazole, administer one IM injection of Abilify Maintena® 400 mg in either the deltoid or gluteal muscle and continue treatment with oral aripiprazole (10–20 mg) for 14 consecutive days to achieve therapeutic aripiprazole concentrations during initiation of therapy For patients already stable on another oral antipsychotic (and known to tolerate aripiprazole), administer one IM injection of Abilify Maintena® 400 mg in either the deltoid or gluteal muscle and continue treatment with the oral antipsychotic for 14 consecutive days to maintain therapeutic antipsychotic concentrations during initiation of therapy
Oral overlap	14 days if not using the 1-day initiation method
Target dose	400 mg IM monthly
Maximum dose	400 mg monthly (no sooner than 26 days after the previous injection)
Dosing interval	Once monthly
Renal/hepatic dosing	None noted in the package insert

IM intramuscular

Table 4.2 Dose conversion of oral to LAI [1, 2]

Oral dose	LAI dose
15 mg aripiprazole	300 mg Abilify Maintena®
20 mg aripiprazole	400 mg Abilify Maintena®

LAI long-acting injectable antipsychotic medication

Table 4.3 Missed dose recommendations [1]

Time from last dose	How to manage
8–12 weeks (i.e., the second or third dose is missed)	If >4 weeks and <5 weeks have elapsed, administer the next injection as soon as possible. If >5 weeks have elapsed, restart treatment with either 1-day initiation or 14-day initiation with Abilify Maintena®.
>12 weeks (i.e., fourth or subsequent doses are missed)	If >4 weeks and <6 weeks have elapsed, administer the injection as soon as possible. If >6 weeks have elapsed, restart treatment with either 1-day initiation or 14-day initiation with Abilify Maintena®.

Table 4.4 Pharmacokinetic Properties [1, 3, 4]

Half-life	Mean apparent terminal elimination half-life: 17.8 days and 21 days, for deltoid and gluteal injections, respectively After multiple gluteal administrations, the mean apparent terminal elimination half-life: 29.9 days and 46.5 days for every 4-week injection of Abilify Maintena® 300 mg and 400 mg, respectively
TMax	5–7 days
Time to steady state	Fourth once-monthly dose
Therapeutic window	100–350 ng/mL

TMax time to maximum concentration

Pharmacokinetic Properties

With its low solubility, aripiprazole particles, following the intramuscular injection, are absorbed into the systemic circulation slowly. The maximum plasma aripiprazole concentrations are reached in approximately 5–7 days. Steady-state aripiprazole concentrations are typically achieved by the fourth once-monthly dose. Table 4.4 provides pharmacokinetic properties of Abilify Maintena® [1, 3, 4].

Drug Interactions

Dosage modifications are recommended for patients who are CYP2D6 poor metabolizers and/or for patients taking concomitant CYP3A4 inhibitors or CYP2D6 inhibitors for more than 14 days. If the CYP3A4 inhibitor or CYP2D6 inhibitor is discontinued, Abilify Maintena® may need to be increased to the previous dose. Concomitant use of CYP3A4 inducers with Abilify Maintena® for greater than 14 days should be avoided, as the blood levels of aripiprazole will be decreased and may be below effective levels. Dosage modifications are not recommended for patients with concomitant use of CYP3A4 inhibitors, CYP2D6 inhibitors, or CYP3A4 inducers for less than 14 days. Tables 4.5 and 4.6 provide details on how to manage drug interactions for both the 1-day and 14-day initiation regimens [1].

Table 4.5 Dosage modifications for Abilify Maintena® (1-day initiation) in patients who are CYP2D6 poor metabolizers and patients taking concomitant CYP2D6 inhibitors, CYP3A4 inhibitors, and/or CYP3A4 inducers for more than 14 days [1]

Metabolizer status	Adjusted dose to be administered[a]
CYP2D6 poor metabolizers	
Known CYP2D6 poor metabolizer	300 mg
Known CYP2D6 poor metabolizer taking concomitant CYP3A4 inhibitor	Avoid use
Concomitant use with CYP inhibitors and/or inducers	
CYP2D6 or CYP3A4 inhibitors	300 mg
CYP2D6 and CYP3A4 inhibitors	Avoid use
CYP3A4 inducers	Avoid use

[a]No change for oral dosage required during initiation

Table 4.6 Dosage modifications for Abilify Maintena® (14-day initiation) in patients who are CYP2D6 poor metabolizers and patients taking concomitant CYP2D6 inhibitors, CYP3A4 Inhibitors, and/or CYP3A4 Inducers for more than 14 days [1]

Metabolizer status	Adjusted dose to be administered[a]
CYP2D6 poor metabolizers	
Known CYP2D6 poor metabolizers	300 mg
Known CYP2D6 poor metabolizers taking concomitant CYP3A4 inhibitors	200 mg
Patients taking 400 mg of Ability Maintena®	
Strong CYP2D6 or CYP3A4 inhibitors	300 mg
CYP2D6 and CYP3A4 inhibitors	200 mg
CYP3A4 inducers	Avoid use
Patients taking 300 mg of Abilify Maintena®	
Strong CYP2D6 or CYP3A4 inhibitors	200 mg
CYP2D6 and CYP3A4 inhibitors	160 mg
CYP3A4 inducers	Avoid use

[a]No change for oral dosage required during initiation

Adverse Effects

Abilify Maintena® is generally well-tolerated with similar adverse effects as the oral aripiprazole products. The most common adverse effects associated with Abilify Maintena® are weight gain, akathisia, insomnia, and injection-site pain. The same warnings and contraindications for aripiprazole oral formulation apply to Ability Maintena® [5–7].

Preparation and Administration Instructions

Abilify Maintena® is available as a prefilled chamber syringe and single-dose vial. The prefilled chamber syringes are 300 and 400 mg strengths, and the single-dose vials are also 300 and 400 mg strengths.

Both the prefilled syringes and single-dose vials should be stored at room temperature. The prefilled syringes should be protected from light by storing them in the original package until the time of administration. Table 4.7 provides details on the injection volumes for the various strengths of Abilify Maintena®.

Injection site: Gluteal or deltoid muscle (rotate the injection site between the two deltoid or gluteal muscles)

Administration instructions:

- Must be administered as intramuscular injection by a health-care professional. Do not administer by any other route.
- As a universal precaution, hands should be washed with soap and water prior to preparation and administration. Gloves should always be worn.

Reconstitution of Lyophilized Powder in Prefilled Dual Chamber Syringe [1]

- Push the plunger rod slightly to engage the threads. Rotate the plunger rod until the rod stops rotating to release the diluent. After the plunger rod is at a complete stop, the middle stopper will be at the indicator line.
- Vertically shake the syringe vigorously for 20 seconds until the medication is uniformly milky white.
- The syringe should not have particulate matter or discoloration prior to administration. The reconstituted product should appear to be a uniform, homogeneous suspension that is opaque and milky-white in color. The injection should be administered within 30 minutes after reconstitution.
- Injection procedure
  - Twist and pull off the over-cap and tip-cap.
  - Select the appropriate needle size. Table 4.8 provides details on which needle size to select for the various body types and injection sites.
  - Ensure the needle is firmly on the safety device with a push. Twist clockwise until snugly fitted.
  - Hold the syringe upright and advance the plunger rod slowly to expel the air. Expel air until suspension fills the needle base.
  - If it's not possible to advance the plunger rod to expel the air, check the plunger rod to verify it is rotated to a complete stop.

Table 4.7 Injection volume [1]

Medication strength (mg)	Injection volume (mL)
160	0.8
200	1
300	1.5
400	2.0

Table 4.8 Needle selection for prefilled syringes [1]

Body type	Injection site	Needle size
Nonobese	Deltoid	1 inch (23 G)
	Gluteus	1.5 inch (22 G)
Obese	Deltoid	1.5 inch (22 G)
	Gluteus	2 inches (21 G)

Table 4.9 Volume of sterile water for injection [1]

400 mg vial		300 mg vial	
Dose	Sterile water for injection	Dose	Sterile water for injection
400 mg	1.9 mL	300 mg	1.5 mL

- Inject the medication slowly. Do not massage the injection site.
- Dispose of the syringe in an appropriate sharps container.

Vial: Preparation and Administration Instructions [1]

- Lay out and confirm that all components that are needed are available and ready for use.
- Only use the sterile water for injection as supplied in the Abilify Maintena® kit.
- Use appropriate aseptic techniques throughout the reconstitution and reconstitute the product at room temperature.
- Select the appropriate amount of sterile water for injection needed for the reconstitution. Table 4.9 provides details on the volume of sterile water for injection to use for reconstitution of the vial.
- Discard any unused portion of the sterile water.

Reconstitution of Lyophilized Powder in Vial [1]

- Remove the cap of the vial of sterile water for injection and remove the cap of the vial containing the powder. Wipe the tops with a sterile alcohol swab.
- Using the syringe with a preattached hypodermic safety needle, withdraw the predetermined sterile water for injection volume from the vial of sterile water for injection into the syringe. Discard any used portion of the sterile water.
- Slowly inject sterile water into the vial containing the powder.
- Withdraw air to equalize the pressure in the vial by pulling back slightly on the plunger. Remove the needle from the vial.
- Shake the vial vigorously for 30 seconds until the reconstituted suspension appears uniform.
- Visually inspect the reconstituted suspension for particulate matter and discoloration prior to administration.
- If the injection is not performed immediately after reconstitution, keep the vial at room temperature. Shake the vial vigorously for at least 60 seconds to resuspend the medication prior to injection.
- Do not store the reconstituted suspension in the syringe.

Preparation Prior to Injection [1]

- Use appropriate aseptic techniques throughout the injection of medication.
- Remove the cover from the vial adapter package. Do not remove the vial adapter from the package.
- Using the vial adapter package to handle the vial adapter, attach the prepackaged Luer lock syringe to the vial adapter.
- Use the Luer lock syringe to remove the vial adapter from the package and discard the vial adapter package. Do not touch the tip of the adapter at any time.
- Determine the recommended volume for injection. Table 4.10 provides details on the injection volume when utilizing the vial.

- Wipe the top of the vial of the reconstituted suspension with a sterile alcohol swab.
- Place and hold the vial of reconstituted suspension on a hard surface. Attach the adapter-syringe assembly to the vial by holding the outside of the adapter and pushing the adapter's spike firmly through the rubber stopper until the adapter snaps in place.
- Slowly withdraw the recommended volume from the vial into the Luer lock syringe to allow for injection. A small amount of excess product will remain in the vial.

Injection Procedure [1]

- Detach the Luer lock syringe containing the recommended volume of medication from the vial.
- Select the appropriate hypodermic safety needle and attach the needle to the Luer lock syringe containing the suspension for injection. Ensure the needle is firmly seated on the safety device with a push. Twist clockwise until snugly fit and then pull the needle cap straight away from the needle. Table 4.11 provides details on the needle size for the different body types and injection sites.

Table 4.10 Injection volume for vials [1]

400 mg vial		300 mg vial	
Dose	Volume to inject	Dose	Volume to inject
400 mg	2 mL	–	–
300 mg	1.5 mL	300 mg	1.5 mL
200 mg	1 mL	200 mg	1 mL
160 mg	0.8 mL	160 mg	0.8 mL

Table 4.11 Needle selection for vials [1]

Body type	Injection site	Needle size
Nonobese	Deltoid	1 inch (23 G)
	Gluteus	1.5 inch (22 G)
Obese	Deltoid	1.5 inch (22 G)
	Gluteus	2 inches (21 G)

- Slowly inject the recommended volume as a single IM injection. Do not massage the injection site.
- Dispose of the syringe in an appropriate sharps container.

References

1. Abilify Maintena® [package insert]. Tokyo: Otsuka Pharmaceutical Co., Ltd.; 2025.
2. VA Pharmacy Benefits Management Services. Aripiprazole long-acting-injection (Abilify Maintena, Aristada) [National Drug Monograph]. 2016.
3. Schoretsanitis G, Bauman P, Conca A, et al. Therapeutic drug monitoring of long-acting injectable antipsychotic drugs. Ther Drug Monit. 2021;43:79–102.
4. Croxtall JD. Aripiprazole: a review of its use in the management of schizophrenia in adults. CNS Drugs. 2012;26:155–83.
5. Kane JM, Sanchez R, Perry PP, et al. Aripiprazole intramuscular depot as maintenance treatment in patients with schizophrenia: a 52-week, multicenter, randomized, double-blind, placebo-controlled study. J Clin Psychiatry. 2012;73:617–24.
6. Fleischhacker WW, Sanchez R, Perry PP, et al. Aripiprazole once-monthly for the treatment of schizophrenia: a double-blind randomized non-inferiority study. Br J Psychiatry. 2014;205(2):135–44.
7. Fleishhacker WW, Sanchez R, Johnson B, et al. Long-term safety and tolerability of aripiprazole once-monthly in maintenance treatment of patients with schizophrenia. Int Clin Psychopharmacol. 2013;28:171–6.

Chapter 5
Aripiprazole Monohydrate (Abilify Asimtufii®): Second-Generation Antipsychotic Long-Acting Injectable

LAI Technology

Abilify Asimtufii® is a lyophilized powder of unmodified aripiprazole, which is constituted in sterile water to an aqueous suspension. Due to the low solubility of the aripiprazole particles, following intramuscular (IM) injection, aripiprazole is absorbed into the systemic circulation slowly [1].

Abilify Asimtufii® is an atypical antipsychotic indicated for the treatment of schizophrenia in adults and as maintenance monotherapy treatment of bipolar I disorder in adults [1].

Dosing Parameters

As with all long-acting injectables (LAIs), establishment of tolerability with prior oral administration is recommended prior to utilization of the long-acting injectable (LAI) formulation. It has been noted that it may take up to 14 days to complete the tolerability testing due to the long half-life of aripiprazole (i.e., 75 h and 94 h for aripiprazole and dehydro-aripiprazole, respectively). Table 5.1 provides dosing recommendations for Abilify Asimtufii® [1].

Abilify Asimtufii® has an established conversion of the oral formulation to the LAI formulation. Table 5.2 provides details on the dose conversion of oral aripiprazole to Abilify Asimtufii® [1].

If an individual misses a scheduled injection of Abilify Asimtufii®, an established missed dose schedule is provided within the package labeling. Table 5.3 provides clinical recommendations on how to manage missed doses of Abilify Asimtufii® [1].

M. J. Ehret, *Long-Acting Injectable Medications in Mental Health*,
https://doi.org/10.1007/978-3-032-09415-5_5

Table 5.1 Dosing recommendations [1]

Initial dose	1-day initiation: Administer 1 IM injection of Abilify Asimtufii® 960 mg in the gluteal muscle, 1 injection of Abilify Maintena® 400 mg in a separate gluteal or deltoid muscle, and one dose of oral aripiprazole 20 mg, on the first day of treatment with Abilify Asimtufii®. Do not administer both injections into the same muscle. 14-day initiation: Administer 1 IM of Abilify Asimtufii® 960 mg in the gluteal muscle and continue treatment with oral aripiprazole (10–20 mg) for 14 consecutive days. Patients already stable on another oral antipsychotic (and known to tolerate aripiprazole), administer 1 IM injection of Abilify Asimtufii® 960 mg in the gluteal muscle and continue treatment with oral antipsychotic for 14 consecutive days. For patients receiving Abilify Maintena® 400 mg (once monthly dosing), administer Abilify Asimtufii® 960 mg (once every 2 months) in place of the next scheduled injection of Abilify Maintena®. The first Abilify Asimtufii® injection may be administered in place of the second or later injection of Abilify Maintena®.
Oral overlap	14 days if not utilizing the 1-day initiation or the patient is not already receiving Abilify Maintena®
Target dose	960 mg administered once every 2 months
Maximum dose	960 mg administered once every 2 months
Dosing interval	Every 8 weeks Patients may be given the Abilify Asimtufii® injection up to 2 weeks before or 2 weeks after the 2-month scheduled timepoint
Renal/hepatic Dosing	None noted in the package insert

IM intramuscular

Table 5.2 Dose conversion of oral to LAI [1]

Oral daily dose	LAI dose
10–20 mg aripiprazole	960 mg Abilify Asimtufii®

LAI long-acting injectable antipsychotic medication

Table 5.3 Missed dose recommendations

Time from last dose	How to manage
>8 weeks and <14 weeks	Administer the next dose of Abilify Asimtufii® as soon as possible; once every 2-month schedule should be resumed
>14 weeks	Restart treatment with either 1-day initiation or 14-day initiation with Abilify Asimtufii®

Pharmacokinetic Properties

Abilify Asimtufii® plasma concentrations following the fourth administration of the injection are similar to the seventh or eighth administration of Abilify Maintena®. Table 5.4 provides pharmacokinetic properties of Abilify Asimtufii® [1, 2].

Table 5.4 Pharmacokinetic properties [1, 2]

Half-life	Mean apparent terminal elimination half-life is 21 days
TMax	1–49 days following multiple gluteal administrations of 960 mg
Time to steady state	Second injection
Therapeutic window	100–350 ng/mL

TMax time to maximum concentration

Table 5.5 Dosage modifications for Abilify Asimtufii® in patients who are CYP2D6 poor metabolizers, patients taking concomitant CYP2D6 inhibitors, CYP3A4 inhibitors, or CYP3A4 inducers for more than 14 days [1]

Metabolizer status	Adjusted dose to be administered
CYP2D6 poor metabolizers	
Known CYP2D6 poor metabolizers	720 mg once every 2 months*
Known CYP2D6 poor metabolizers taking concomitant CYP3A4 inhibitors	Avoid use
Patients taking 960 mg of Abilify Asimtufii®	
Concomitant use of Abilify Asimtufii® with strong CYP2D6 inhibitors	720 mg once every 2 months*
Concomitant use of Abilify Asimtufii® with strong CYP3A4 inhibitors	720 mg once every 2 months*
Concomitant use of Abilify Asimtufii® with strong CYP2D6 and strong CYP3A4 inhibitors	Avoid use
Concomitant use of Abilify Asimtufii® with CYP3A4 inducers	Avoid use

*For the 1-day initiation regimen, administer a single 20 mg oral aripiprazole, 300 mg Abilify Maintena®, and 720 mg Abilify Asimtufii® on Day 1.

Drug Interactions

Dosage modifications are recommended for patients who are CYP2D6 poor metabolizers and/or in patients taking concomitant CYP3A4 inhibitors or CYP2D6 inhibitors for more than 14 days. If the CYP3A4 inhibitor or CYP2D6 inhibitor is discontinued, Abilify Asimtufii® may need to be increased to the previous dose. Dosage modifications are not recommended for patients with concomitant use of CYP3A4 inhibitors, CYP2D6 inhibitors, or CYP3A4 inducers for less than 14 days. Table 5.5 provides details on how to manage drug interactions for Abilify Asimtufii® [1].

Adverse Reactions

Abilify Asimtufii® is generally well tolerated with similar adverse effects as the oral aripiprazole products. The most common adverse effects were weight gain, akathisia, insomnia, and injection-site pain. The same warnings and contraindications for aripiprazole oral formulation apply to Abilify Asimtufii® [3].

Preparation and Administration Instructions

Abilify Asimtufii® is available as a prefilled syringe available as 720 and 960 mg strengths. These syringes should be stored at room temperature. Table 5.6 provides details on the injection volume [1].

Injection site: Gluteal muscle (rotate the site of injection between the two gluteal muscles)

Administration instructions [1]:

- Must be administered as intramuscular injections by a health-care professional. Do not administer by any other route.
- As a universal precaution, hands should be washed with soap and water prior to preparation and administration. Gloves should always be worn.
- Visually inspect the prefilled syringe for particulate matter and discoloration. The suspension should appear uniform, homogeneous, opaque, and milky white in color.
- Remove the prefilled syringe from the package.
- Tap the syringe on your hand at least ten times.
- After tapping, shake the syringe vigorously for at least 10 seconds, until the medication is uniform.
- Select the appropriate needle size. Table 5.7 provides details on the needle size for various body types.
- Attach the needle by twisting and pulling off the prefilled syringe tip-cap and gently twisting the needle clockwise until securely fitted.
- Hold the prefilled syringe upright and remove the needle-cap straight up.

Table 5.6 Injection volume [1]

Medication strength (mg)	Injection volume (mL)
720	2.4
960	3.2

Table 5.7 Needle size selection [1]

Body type	Needle size
Nonobese	1.5 inch (22 G)
Obese	2 inches (21 G)

- Slowly advance the plunger rod upward to expel the air until the suspension fills the needle base.
- Slowly inject the entire contents of the prefilled syringe. Do not massage the injection site.
- Dispose of needle in appropriate sharps container.

References

1. Abilify Asimtufii® [package insert]. Tokyo: Otsuka, Pharmaceutical Co., Ltd.; 2025.
2. Schoretsanitis G, Bauman P, Conca A, et al. Therapeutic drug monitoring of long-acting injectable antipsychotic drugs. Ther Drug Monit. 2021;43:79–102.
3. Harlin M, Yildirim M, Such P, et al. A randomized, open-label, multiple-dose, parallel-arm, pivotal study to evaluate the safety, tolerability, and pharmacokinetics of aripiprazole 2-month long-acting injectable in adults with schizophrenia or bipolar I disorder. CNS Drugs. 2023;24:337–50.

Chapter 6
Aripiprazole Lauroxil (Aristada®): Second-Generation Antipsychotic Long-Acting Injectable

LAI Technology

Aristada® utilizes LinkRx® technology, which has a linker to attach aripiprazole to a fatty acid tail to form aripiprazole Lauroxil. This attachment allows for lower solubility of aripiprazole for controlled release after each injection and extends exposure to the active molecule. An enzyme-mediated cleavage by esterases cleaves the fatty acid from the linker. The linker then reacts with the water to leave free aripiprazole [1].

Aristada® is an atypical antipsychotic indicated for the treatment of schizophrenia in adults [2].

Dosing Parameters

As with all long-acting injectable (LAI) antipsychotics, establishment of tolerability with prior oral administration is recommended prior to utilization of the LAI formulation. It has been noted that it may take up to 14 days to complete the tolerability testing due to the long half-life of aripiprazole (i.e., 75 h and 94 h for aripiprazole and dehydro-aripiprazole, respectively). Table 6.1 provides dosing recommendations for Aristada® [2].

Aristada® has an established conversion of the oral formulation to the LAI formulation. Table 6.2 provides details on the dose conversion from oral aripiprazole to Aristada®.

When a dose is missed, administer the next injection as soon as possible. Depending on the time elapsed since the last Aristada® injection, supplement the next Aristada® injection as recommended in Table 6.3. Table 6.3 provides clinical recommendations on how to manage missed doses of Aristada®.

- In the event of early dosing, Aristada® should not be given earlier than 14 days after the previous injection.

M. J. Ehret, *Long-Acting Injectable Medications in Mental Health*, https://doi.org/10.1007/978-3-032-09415-5_6

Table 6.1 Dosing recommendations [2]

Initial dose	Loading strategy 1: Administer one IM injection of Aristada Initio® 675 mg (in either the deltoid or gluteal muscle) and one dose of oral aripiprazole 30 mg in conjunction with the first Aristada® injection. The first Aristada® injection may be administered on the same day as Aristada Initio® or up to 10 days thereafter. Avoid injecting both Aristada Initio® and Aristada® concomitantly into the same deltoid or gluteal muscle. Loading strategy 2: Administer 21 consecutive days of oral aripiprazole in conjunction with the first Aristada® injection.
Oral overlap	21 days required if not utilizing loading strategy 1
Target dose	Depending on the patient's oral dose, Aristada® can be initiated at a dose of 441 mg, 662 mg, or 882 mg administered monthly, 882 mg administered every 6 weeks, or 1064 mg administered every 8 weeks.
Maximum dose	882 mg every 4 weeks
Dosing interval	Every 4, 6, or 8 weeks, depending on the needs of the patient
Renal/hepatic dosing	None noted in the package insert

IM intramuscular

Table 6.2 Dose conversion of oral to LAI [2]

Oral daily dose	LAI dose
10 mg aripiprazole	441 mg Aristada® every 4 weeks
15 mg aripiprazole	662 mg Aristada® every 4 weeks 882 mg Aristada® every 6 weeks 1064 mg Aristada® every 8 weeks
20 mg or higher aripiprazole	882 mg Aristada® every 4 weeks

LAI long-acting injectable antipsychotic medication

Table 6.3 Missed dose recommendations [2]

Dose of patient's last Aristada® injection	Length of time since the last injection		
441 mg	≤6 weeks	>6 and ≤7 weeks	>7 weeks
662 mg	≤8 weeks	>8 and ≤12 weeks	>12 weeks
882 mg	≤8 weeks	>8 weeks and ≤12 weeks	>12 weeks
1064 mg	≤10 weeks	>10 and ≤12 weeks	>12 weeks
Dosage and administration for reinitiation of Aristada®	No supplementation required	Supplement with a single dose of Aristada Initio® or 7 days of oral aripiprazole[a]	Reinitiate with a single dose of Aristada Initio® and a single dose of oral aripiprazole 30 mg, or supplement with 21 days of oral aripiprazole[a]

[a]The same dose of oral aripiprazole as when the patient began Aristada®

Table 6.4 Pharmacokinetic properties [2, 3]

Half-life	Mean aripiprazole terminal elimination half-life ranges from 53.9 to 57.2 days after monthly, every 6-week, and every 2-month injections
TMax	With Aristada Initio® loading strategy 1: 4 days Without Aristada Initio® loading strategy: 54–57 days
Time to steady state	Fourth monthly injection
Therapeutic window	100–350 ng/mL

TMax time to maximum concentration

Pharmacokinetic Properties

Systemic absorption of aripiprazole following a single intramuscular injection occurs within 5–6 days and continues to be released for an additional 36 days. Concentrations® of the medication continue to build and will reach a steady state following the fourth monthly administration. Table 6.4 provides details on the pharmacokinetic properties of Aristada®.

Drug Interactions

For the first 21 days, if the patient is receiving oral aripiprazole, the prescriber should refer to the prescribing information for oral aripiprazole for recommendations on dosage. Aristada® use with Aristada Initio® should be avoided in patients requiring dose adjustments. Once the patient is stabilized on Aristada®, dosing recommendations are available for patients taking strong CYP2D6 inhibitors, strong CYP3A4 inhibitors, or strong CYP3A4 inducers. There are no dosage change recommendations for Aristada® if CYP450 modulators are added for less than 2 weeks. If CYP450 modulators are added for greater than 14 days, Table 6.5 provides detailed recommendations. Table 6.5 provides details on how to manage drug interactions.

Table 6.5 Aristada® dose adjustments with concomitant CYP450 modulators [2]

Concomitant medication	Dose change recommendation for Aristada[a]
Strong CYP3A4 inhibitor	Reduce the dose of Aristada® to the next lower strength. No dosage adjustment is necessary in patients taking 441 mg Aristada®, if tolerated. For patients known to be poor metabolizers of CYP2D6: Reduce dose to 441 mg from 662 mg, 882, or 1064 mg. No dosage adjustment is necessary in patients taking 441 mg Aristada®, if tolerated.
Strong CYP2D6 inhibitor	Reduce the dose of Aristada® to the next lower strength. No dosage adjustment is necessary in patients taking 441 mg Aristada®, if tolerated. For patients known to be poor metabolizers of CYP2D6: No dose adjustment is required.
Both a strong CYP3A4 inhibitor and a strong CYP2D6 inhibitor	Avoid use for patients at 662 mg, 882 mg, or 1064 mg doses. No dose adjustment is necessary in patients taking 441 mg Aristada®, if tolerated.
CYP3A4 inducers	No dose adjustment for 662 mg, 882 mg, or 1064 mg doses; increase the 441 mg dose to 662 mg.

[a]For the 882 mg dose administered every 6 weeks and the 1064 mg administered every 2 months, the next lower strength should be 441 mg administered monthly

Adverse Reactions

Aristada® is generally well-tolerated with similar adverse effects as the oral aripiprazole products. The most common adverse effects were weight gain, akathisia, insomnia, and injection-site pain. The same warnings and contraindications for aripiprazole oral formulation are applicable to Aristada® [1].

Preparation and Administration Instructions

Aristada® is available as a prefilled syringe in 441, 662, 882, and 1064 mg strengths. These syringes should be stored at room temperature. The boxes of prefilled syringes should be stored flat to avoid clogging when administering the medication. Table 6.6 provides details on the injection volume [2].

Injection site: Gluteal muscle (all doses) and deltoid muscle (441 mg dose only)

Administration instructions [2]:

- Must be administered as intramuscular injections by a healthcare professional. Do not administer by any other route.

Table 6.6 Injection volume [2]

Medication strength (mg)	Injection volume (mL)
441	1.6
662	2.4
882	3.2
1064	3.9

Table 6.7 Needle size selection [2]

Injection site	Needle length[a]
441 mg dose	
Deltoid	1 inch (21 G) 1.5 inch (20 G)
Gluteal	1.5 inch (20 G) 2 inches (20 G)
662 mg dose	
Gluteal	1.5 inch (20 G) 2 inches (20 G)
882 mg dose	
Gluteal	1.5 inch (20 G) 2 inches (20 G)
1064 mg dose	
Gluteal	1.5 inch (20 G) 2 inches (20 G)

[a]For patients with a larger amount of subcutaneous tissue overlaying the injection site muscle, use the longer of the needles

- As a universal precaution, hands should be washed with soap and water prior to preparation and administration. Gloves should always be worn.
- Tap the syringe at least 10 times to dislodge any material that may have settled.
- Shake the syringe vigorously for a minimum of 30 seconds to ensure uniform suspension. If the syringe is not used within 15 minutes, shake again for 30 seconds.
- Select the injection needle and injection site. Table 6.7 provides details on the needle size for the various doses and injection sites.
- Attach the injection needle with a clockwise twisting motion. Do not overtighten, which could lead to needle hub cracking.
- Prime the syringe to remove air.
- Bring the syringe into an upright position and tap the syringe to bring air to the top.
- Depress the plunger rod to remove air until a few drops are released. It is normal to see small air bubbles remaining in the syringe.
- Inject in a rapid and continuous manner. The product requires rapid injection. Do not hesitate. Administer the entire content intramuscularly.
- Dispose of the syringe in an appropriate sharps container.

References

1. Cruz MP. Aripiprazole Lauroxil (Aristada). PT. 2016;41:556–9.
2. Aristada® [package insert]. Waltham: Alkermes, Inc.; 2025.
3. Schoretsanitis G, Bauman P, Conca A, et al. Therapeutic drug monitoring of long-acting injectable antipsychotic drugs. Ther Drug Monit. 2021;43:79–102.

Chapter 7
Aripiprazole Lauroxil Nanocrystal Technology (Aristada Initio®): Second-Generation Antipsychotic

LAI Technology

Aristada Initio® is composed of a nanometer-sized particles, with a surface area-to-volume ratio up to 1000 times larger than its micrometer counterpart. This results in a faster rise in plasma medication levels after administration, earlier peak plasma levels, and a shorter half-life than a formulation with a larger particle size [1]. Aristada Initio® also utilizes LinkRx® technology, which has a linker to attach aripiprazole to a fatty acid tail to form aripiprazole lauroxil. This attachment allows for lower solubility of aripiprazole for controlled release after each injection and extends exposure to the active molecule. An enzyme-mediated cleavage by esterases cleaves the fatty acid from the linker. The linker then reacts with the water to leave free aripiprazole [1].

Aristada Initio®, in combination with oral aripiprazole, is indicated for the initiation of Aristada® when used for the treatment of schizophrenia in adults [2].

Dosing Parameters

As with all long-acting injectables (LAIs), establishment of tolerability with prior oral administration is recommended prior to utilization of this initiation formulation. It has been noted that it may take up to 14 days to complete the tolerability testing due to the long half-life of aripiprazole (i.e., 75 h and 94 h for aripiprazole and dehydro-aripiprazole, respectively) [2].

Aristada Initio® is only to be used as a single dose to initiate Aristada® treatment or as a single dose to reinitiate Aristada® treatment following a missed dose of Aristada®. Aristada® is not for repeated dosing. After establishing tolerability with oral aripiprazole, administer the first Aristada® intramuscular injection (441 mg,

M. J. Ehret, *Long-Acting Injectable Medications in Mental Health*,
https://doi.org/10.1007/978-3-032-09415-5_7

Table 7.1 Missed dose recommendations [1]

Dose of patient's last Aristada® injection	Length of time since last injection		
441 mg	≤6 weeks	>6 and ≤7 weeks	>7 weeks
662 mg	≤8 weeks	>8 and ≤12 weeks	>12 weeks
882 mg	≤8 weeks	>8 weeks and ≤12 weeks	>12 weeks
1064 mg	≤10 weeks	>10 and ≤12 weeks	>12 weeks
Dosage and administration for reinitiation of Aristada®	No supplementation required	Supplement with a single dose of Aristada Initio®	Reinitiate with a single dose of Aristada Initio® and a single dose of oral aripiprazole 30 mg

662 mg, 882 mg, or 1064 mg) in conjunction with both one 675 mg injection of Aristada Initio® in the deltoid or gluteal muscle and one 30 mg dose of oral aripiprazole [2].

The first Aristada® injection may be administered on the same day as Aristada Initio® or up to 10 days thereafter. Avoid injecting Aristada Initio® and Aristada® concomitantly into the same deltoid or gluteal muscle [2].

If an individual misses a scheduled injection of Aristada®, an established missed dose schedule has been provided within the package insert. Table 7.1 provides details on how to manage a missed dose. Table 7.2 provides details on the pharmacokinetic properties of Aristada Initio® [2].

Pharmacokinetic Properties

Table 7.2 Pharmacokinetic properties [2]

Half-life	Mean aripiprazole terminal elimination half-life: 15–18 days after injection
TMax	In combination with 30 mg tablet: 4 days Without combination with 30 mg tablet: 16–35 days

TMax time to maximum concentration

Drug Interactions

This medication is only available as a single 675 mg dose, so dosage adjustments are not possible. Patients who are CYP2D6 poor metabolizers or are taking strong CYP3A4 inhibitors, strong CYP2D6 inhibitors, or strong CYP3A4 inducers should avoid use [2].

Adverse Reactions

Aristada Initio® is generally well-tolerated with similar adverse effects as the oral aripiprazole products. The most common adverse effects were weight gain, akathisia, insomnia, and injection-site pain. The same warnings and contraindications for aripiprazole oral formulation are applicable to Aristada Initio® [2].

Preparation and Administration Instructions

Aristada Initio® is available as a prefilled syringe available in 675 mg strength. These prefilled syringes should be stored at room temperature. The boxes of syringes should be stored flat to avoid clogging [2].

Injection site: Gluteal or deltoid muscle

Injection volume: 2.4 mL

Administration Instructions [2]:

- Must be administered as an intramuscular injection by a health-care professional. Do not administer by any other route.
- As a universal precaution, hands should be washed with soap and water prior to preparation and administration. Gloves should always be worn.
- Tap the syringe at least 10 times to dislodge any material that may have settled.
- Shake the syringe vigorously for a minimum of 30 seconds to ensure uniform suspension. If the syringe is not used within 15 minutes, shake again for 30 seconds.
- Select the needle size and injection site. Table 7.3 provides details on needle size selection based on the injection site.
- Attach the injection needle by twisting clockwise. Do not overtighten, which could lead to needle hub cracking.
- Prime the syringe to remove air.
- Bring the syringe into an upright position and tap the syringe to bring air to the top.
- Depress the plunger rod to remove air until a few drops are released. It is normal to see small air bubbles remaining in the syringe.

Table 7.3 Needle size selection [2]

Injection site	Needle length
675 mg dose	Needle length[a]
Deltoid	1 inch (21 G) 1.5 inch (20 G)
Gluteal	1.5 inch (20 G) 2 inches (20 G)

[a]For patients with a larger amount of subcutaneous tissue overlaying the injection site muscle, use the longer of the needles

- Inject in a rapid and continuous manner. The medication required a rapid injection. Do not hesitate. Administer the entire content intramuscularly.
- Dispose of syringe in appropriate sharps container.

References

1. Jain R, Meyer J, Wehr A, et al. Size matters: the importance of particle size in a newly developed injectable formulation for the treatment of schizophrenia. CNS Spectr. 2020;25:323–30.
2. Aristada Initio® [package insert]. Waltham: Alkermes, Inc.; 2025.

Chapter 8
Paliperidone Palmitate (Invega Sustenna®): Second-Generation Antipsychotic Long-Acting Injectable

LAI Technology

Intramuscular paliperidone palmitate is the palmitate ester of paliperidone. The injection contains a nanocrystal molecule in an aqueous solution, which has very low water solubility. It dissolves slowly after intramuscular injection [1]. The medication is then hydrolyzed by esterases in muscle tissue to its major active metabolite, paliperidone, and absorbed systemically [2].

Invega Sustenna® is an atypical antipsychotic indicated for the treatment of schizophrenia in adults and schizoaffective disorder in adults as monotherapy and as an adjunct to mood stabilizers or antidepressants [3].

Dosing Parameters

As with all long-acting injectable (LAIs), establishment of tolerability with prior oral administration is recommended prior to utilization of the LAI formulation. Table 8.1 provides dosing recommendations for Invega Sustenna® [3].

Invega Sustenna® has an established conversion of the oral formulation to the LAI formulation. Table 8.2 provides the dose conversion from oral paliperidone to Invega Sustenna®. Dose conversions from oral risperidone to Invega Sustenna® have been developed based on pharmacokinetic modeling: 1 mg = 39 mg of the LAI, 2 mg = 78 mg of the LAI, 3 mg = 117 mg of the LAI®, 4 mg = 156 mg of the LAI, and 6 mg = 234 mg of the LAI [4]. Table 8.3 provides details on dose conversions of Risperdal Consta® to Invega Sustenna®.

If an individual should miss a scheduled injection of Invega Sustenna®, an established missed dose schedule has been established within the package insert. Table 8.4 provides details on how to manage a missed second initiation dose of

M. J. Ehret, *Long-Acting Injectable Medications in Mental Health*,
https://doi.org/10.1007/978-3-032-09415-5_8

Table 8.1 Dosing recommendations [3]

Initial dose	Loading dose: 234 mg on Day 1, followed by 156 mg on Day 8, followed by maintenance dose 5 weeks after first injection[a] (loading dose injections are recommended to be given in the deltoid muscle)
Oral overlap	Not required
Target dose	117 mg monthly
Maximum dose	234 mg monthly
Dosing interval	Every 4 weeks
Renal/hepatic dosing	Mild renal impairment: CrCl ≥50 mL/min to <80 mL/min (Cockcroft-Gault Formula), initiate Invega Sustenna® with a dose of 156 mg on treatment Day 1 and 117 mg on Day 8, both in the deltoid muscle. Follow with the recommended monthly maintenance dose of 78 mg, either deltoid or gluteal. The maximum dose is 156 mg. No hepatic dosing noted in package insert.

IM intramuscular, *CrCl* creatine clearance
[a]Second loading injection can be given 4 days before or after the 1-week time point

Table 8.2 Dose conversion of oral to LAI paliperidone [3]

Oral daily dose	LAI dose
3 mg paliperidone	39–78 mg Invega Sustenna®
6 mg paliperidone	117 mg Invega Sustenna®
9 mg paliperidone	156 mg Invega Sustenna®
12 mg paliperidone	234 mg Invega Sustenna®

LAI long-acting injectable antipsychotic medication

Table 8.3 Dose conversion from Risperdal Consta® to Invega Sustenna® [3]

Risperdal Consta® every two-week dose (mg)	Invega Sustenna® injection to be administered in place of the next scheduled injection (mg)[a]
25	78
37.5	117
50	156

[a]Patients may benefit from lower or higher maintenance doses with the full range of Invega Sustenna® dosing

Invega Sustenna®, while Table 8.5 provides details on how to manage a missed maintenance dose.

- When switching patients currently at steady state on a LAI antipsychotic, initiate Invega Sustenna® therapy in place of the next scheduled injection.

Table 8.4 Missed dose recommendations–second initiation dose [3]

Timing of missed second initiation dose	Dosing recommended
<4 weeks since the first injection	Administer the second initiation dose of 156 mg in the deltoid muscle as soon as possible. Administer a third injection of 117 mg in either the deltoid or gluteal muscle 5 weeks after the first injection (regardless of the timing of the second injection). Resume regular monthly dosing in either the deltoid or gluteal muscle.
4–7 weeks since the first injection	Resume dosing with 2 injections of 156 mg in the following manner: Administer a deltoid injection as soon as possible Administer a second deltoid injection 1 week later Resume regular monthly dosing in either the deltoid or gluteal muscle.
>7 weeks since the first injection	Restart dosing with recommended initiation: Administer a 234 mg deltoid injection on Day 1 Administer a 156 mg deltoid injection 1 week later Resume regular monthly dosing in either the deltoid or gluteal muscle.

Table 8.5 Missed dose recommendations–maintenance dose [3]

Timing of missed maintenance dose	Dosing recommendations
4–6 weeks since the last injection	Resume regular monthly dosing as soon as possible at the patient's previously stabilized dose, followed by injections at monthly intervals.
>6 weeks–6 months since the last injection	Resume the same dose the patient was previously stabilized on (unless the patient was stabilized on 234 mg, then the first two injections should each be 156 mg) in the following manner: Administer a deltoid injection as soon as possible Administer a second deltoid injection 1 week later at the same dose Resume administering the previously stabilized dose in the deltoid or gluteal muscle 1 month after the second injection
>6 months since the last injection	Restart dosing with recommended initiation: Administer a 234 mg deltoid injection on Day 1 Administer a 156 mg deltoid injection 1 week later Resume administering the previously stabilized dose in the deltoid or gluteal muscle 1 month after the second injection

Pharmacokinetic Properties

The maximum concentration values are approximately 28% higher after administration of a single dose of intramuscular paliperidone palmitate into the deltoid versus the gluteal muscle. This has led to the recommendation of using the deltoid muscle for the loading doses to rapidly obtain the therapeutic concentrations [1]. The release of the active mediation occurs as early as the first day and lasts ≥4 months. Table 8.6 provides details on the pharmacokinetic properties of Invega Sustenna® [3, 4].

Table 8.6 Pharmacokinetic properties [3, 4]

Half-life	Median apparent half-life ranged 25–49 days
TMax	13 days
Therapeutic window	20–60 ng/mL

TMax time to maximum concentration

Drug Interactions

Invega Sustenna® should be avoided with a strong inducer of CYP3A4 and/or P-glycoprotein medications during the 1-month dosing interval for Invega Sustenna®, if possible. If administering a strong inducer is necessary, consider managing the patient using paliperidone extended-release tablets [3].

Adverse Reactions

Invega Sustenna® is generally well-tolerated with similar adverse effects as the oral paliperidone products. The most common adverse effects were agitation, akathisia, constipation, diarrhea, dizziness, headache, injection-site reactions, insomnia, nausea, somnolence, tachycardia, tremor, and weight gain [5, 6].

Preparation and Administration Instructions

Invega Sustenna® is available as a prefilled syringe in 39, 78, 117, 156, and 234 mg strengths. These syringes should be stored at room temperature. Table 8.7 provides details on the injection volume [3].

Injection site: Deltoid and gluteal muscle (upper-outer quadrant of the gluteal muscle)

Administration instructions [3]:

- Must be administered as an intramuscular injection by a health-care professional. Do not administer by any other route.
- As a universal precaution, hands should be washed with soap and water prior to preparation and administration. Gloves should always be worn.
- Shake the syringe vigorously for a minimum of 10 seconds to ensure a homogeneous suspension.
- Select the appropriate needle and injection site. Table 8.8 provides details on the needle size for the different injection sites.
- Hold the syringe with the tip-cap pointing upward. Remove the rubber tip-cap with a gentle twisting motion.

Table 8.7 Injection volume [3]

Medication strength (mg)	Injection volume (mL)
39	0.25
78	0.5
117	0.75
156	1
234	1.5

Table 8.8 Needle size selection [3]

Injection site	Needle size
Deltoid	Patients weighing <90 kg: 1 inch (23 G) Patients weighing >90 kg or more: 1.5 inch (22 G)
Gluteal	1.5 inch (22 G)

- Peel the safety needle pouch halfway open. Grasp the needle sheath using the plastic peel pouch, and hold the syringe pointing upward. Attach the safety needle to the syringe using a gentle twisting motion to avoid needle hub cracks or damage.
- Pull the needle sheath away from the needle with a straight pull.
- Bring the syringe with the attached needle in an upright position to deaerate. Deaerate the syringe by moving the plunger rod carefully forward.
- Inject the entire contents intramuscularly slowly, deep into the selected deltoid or gluteal muscle.
- Dispose of the syringe in an appropriate sharps container.

References

1. Janssen-Cilag International NV. Paliperidone palmitate 25, 50, 75, 100, and 150 mg prolonged-release suspension for injection (Xeplion®): EU summary of product characteristics [online].
2. Gilday E, Nasrallah HA. Clinical pharmacology of paliperidone palmitate a parenteral long-acting formulation for the treatment of schizophrenia. Rev Recent Clin Trials. 2012;7:2–9.
3. Invega Sustenna® [package insert]. Titusville: Janssen Pharmaceuticals, Inc.; 2025.
4. Russu A, Kern Sliwa J, Ravenstijn P, et al. Maintenance dose conversion between oral risperidone and paliperidone palmitate 1 month: practical guidance based on pharmacokinetic simulations. Int J Clin Pract. 2018;72:e13089.
5. Schoretsanitis G, Bauman P, Conca A, et al. Therapeutic drug monitoring of long-acting injectable antipsychotic drugs. Ther Drug Monit. 2021;43:79–102.
6. Carter N. Extended-release intramuscular paliperidone palmitate. Drugs. 2012;72:1137–60.

Chapter 9
Paliperidone Palmitate (Invega Trinza®): Second-Generation Antipsychotic Long-Acting Injectable

LAI Technology

Invega Trinza® uses a larger particle size than that created for Invega Sustenna® to facilitate a slower release. Peak plasma medication levels are observed at 30–33 days postinjection compared to 7–8 days postinjection for the smaller particle size in Invega Sustenna® [1].

Invega Trinza® is an atypical antipsychotic indicated for the treatment of schizophrenia in patients after being adequately treated with Invega Sustenna® for at least 4 months [2].

Dosing Parameters [2]

- Use Invega Trinza® only after the patient has been adequately treated with 1-month paliperidone palmitate extended-release injectable suspension for at least 4 months. The last 2 months of paliperidone palmitate should be the same dose.
- As with all long-acting injectables (LAIs), establishment of tolerability® with prior oral administration is recommended prior to utilization of the LAI formulation. Table 9.1 provides details on the dosing recommendations for Invega Trinza®.

Invega Trinza® has an established conversion of the oral formulation to the LAI formulation. Table 9.2 provides details on the dose conversion of oral paliperidone to paliperidone palmitate to Invega Trinza® [2].

If an individual misses a scheduled injection of Invega Trinza®, an established missed dose schedule® has been provided within the package insert. Table 9.3 provides details on how to manage a missed dose of Invega Trinza® [2]. Table 9.4

M. J. Ehret, *Long-Acting Injectable Medications in Mental Health*,
https://doi.org/10.1007/978-3-032-09415-5_9

Table 9.1 Dosing recommendations [2]

Initial dose	Based on the dose of Invega Sustenna®
Oral overlap	Not required
Target dose	Based on the dose of Invega Sustenna®
Maximum dose	819 mg every 3 months
Dosing interval	Every 3 months
Renal/hepatic dosing	Mild renal impairment: CrCl ≥50 mL/min–<80 mL/min (Cockcroft-Gault Formula): Adjust dosage and stabilize the patient using paliperidone palmitate, then transition to Invega Trinza®.

IM Intramuscular, *CrCl* Creatine clearance

Table 9.2 Dose conversion of oral to LAI–paliperidone to Invega Trinza® [2]

Oral daily dose	LAI dose paliperidone palmitate	LAI Dose–Invega Trinza® [a]
<3 mg paliperidone	39 mg paliperidone palmitate every 4 weeks	N/A
3 mg paliperidone	78 mg paliperidone palmitate every 4 weeks	273 mg every 12 weeks
6 mg paliperidone	117 mg paliperidone palmitate every 4 weeks	410 mg every 12 weeks
9 mg paliperidone	156 mg paliperidone palmitate every 4 weeks	546 mg every 12 weeks
12 mg paliperidone	234 mg paliperidone palmitate every 4 weeks	819 mg every 12 weeks

LAI Long-acting injectable antipsychotic medication
[a]Patients may be given the injection up to 2 weeks before or after the 3-month time point. Utilizing the flexible dosing window should be considered the exception rather than the rule

Table 9.3 Missed dose recommendations [2]

Time since the last injection	How to manage
3.5–4 months	The previously administered Invega Trinza® dose should be administered as soon as possible, then continue the 3-month injections following the dose.
4–9 months	Do not administer the next dose of Invega Trinza®. Use the following reinitiation table. (Table 9.4)

Table 9.4 Reinitiation regimen after missing 4–9 months of Invega Trinza® [2]

Last dose of Invega Trinza®	Administer these paliperidone palmitate, two doses 1 week apart (into the deltoid muscle)		Then administer Invega Trinza® (into the deltoid or gluteal muscle)
	Day 1	Day 8	1 month after Day 8
273 mg	78 mg	78 mg	273 mg
410 mg	117 mg	117 mg	410 mg
546 mg	156 mg	156 mg	546 mg
819 mg	156 mg	156 mg	819 mg

provides details on how to reinitiate a regimen of Invega Trinza® after missing a dose 4–9 months ago [2]. Table 9.5 provides the pharmacokinetic properties [2, 3].

- If more than 9 months have elapsed since the last injection, reinitiate treatment with the 1-month paliperidone palmitate as described in the prescribing information for that product.

Pharmacokinetic Properties

Table 9.5 Pharmacokinetic properties [3]

Half-life	Median apparent half-life ranges from 84 days to 95 days following deltoid injections and 118–139 days following gluteal injections.
TMax	30–33 days
Therapeutic window	20–60 ng/mL

TMax Time to maximum concentration

Drug Interactions

No specific drug interaction studies were performed with Invega Trinza® [2].

Adverse Reactions

Invega Trinza® is generally well-tolerated with similar adverse effects to the oral paliperidone products. The most common adverse effects were agitation, akathisia, constipation, diarrhea, dizziness, headache, injection-site reactions, insomnia, nausea, somnolence, tachycardia, tremor, and weight gain [4].

Preparation and Administration Instructions

Invega Trinza® is available as a prefilled syringe with 273, 410, 546, and 819 mg strengths. These syringes should be stored at room temperature. Table 9.6 provides details on the injection volume [2].

Injection site: Deltoid or gluteal muscle

Administration instructions [2]:

- Must be administered as an intramuscular injection by a health-care professional. Do not administer by any other route.

Table 9.6 Injection volume [2]

Medication strength	Injection volume
273 mg	0.875 mL
410 mg	1.315 mL
546 mg	1.75 mL
819 mg	2.625 mL

Table 9.7 Needle size selection [2]

Injection site	Needle size
Deltoid	Patients weighing <90 kg: 1 inch (22G) Patients weighing >90 kg or more: 1.5 inch (22G)
Gluteal	Patients weighing <90 kg: 1.5 inch (22G) Patients weighing >90 kg or more: 1.5 inch (22G)

- As a universal precaution, hands should be washed with soap and water prior to preparation and adminsitration. Gloves should always be worn.
- Select the needle and injection site. Table 9.7 provides the needle size selection based on the injection site.
- Shake the prefilled syringe for at least 15 seconds. If more than 5 minutes pass before injection, shake vigorously with the syringe tip pointing upward again for at least 15 seconds to resuspend the medication.
- After shaking the syringe for at least 15 seconds, check the liquid in the viewing window. The suspension should appear uniform and milky white in color. It is also normal to see small air bubbles.
- Open the needle pouch and remove the cap.
- Grasp the needle pouch and attach the needle with a twisting motion to avoid needle hub cracks or damage.
- Remove the needle sheath in a straight motion.
- Hold the syringe upright and tap gently to make air bubbles rise to the top. Remove air by pressing the plunger rod upward carefully until a drop of liquid comes out of the needle tip.
- Slowly inject the entire contents of the syringe intramuscularly, deep into the selected deltoid or gluteal muscle.
- Dispose of the syringe in an appropriate sharps container.

References

1. Jain R, Meyer J, Wehr A, et al. Size matters: the importance of particle size in a newly developed injectable formulation for the treatment of schizophrenia. CNS Spectr. 2020;25:323–30.
2. Invega Trinza® [package insert]. Titusville: Janssen Pharmaceuticals, Inc; 2025.
3. Schoretsanitis G, Bauman P, Conca A, et al. Therapeutic drug monitoring of long-acting injectable antipsychotic drugs. Ther Drug Monit. 2021;43:79–102.
4. Lopez A, Rey J. Role of paliperidone palmitate 3-monthly in the management of schizophrenia: insights from clinical practice. Neuropsychiatr Dis Treat. 2019;15:449–56.

Chapter 10
Paliperidone Palmitate (Invega Hafyera®): Second-Generation Antipsychotic Long-Acting Injectable

LAI Technology

Invega Hafyera® uses a larger particle size than that created for Invega Trinza® to facilitate a slower release. The release of the medication starts as early as day one and is predicted to last longer than 18 months [1].

Invega Hafyera® is an atypical antipsychotic indicated for the treatment of schizophrenia in adults who have been adequately treated with a once-monthly paliperidone palmitate for at least 4 months or an every 3-month Invega Trinza® for at least one 3-month cycle [1].

Dosing Parameters

- Initiate Invega Hafyera® when the next once-a-month or every 3-month paliperidone palmitate extended-release injectable suspension dose is scheduled. Dose is based on the previous once-a-month or every 3-month product [1].
- Table 10.1 provides the dosing recommendations for Invega Hafyera®.
  - Invega Hafyera® may be administered up to 1 week before or 1 week after the next scheduled paliperidone palmitate dose.
  - Invega Hafyera® may be administered up to 2 weeks before or 2 weeks after the next scheduled Invega Trinza® dose.

Invega Hafyera® has an established conversion from paliperidone palmitate and Invega Trinza® to Invega Hafyera®. Table 10.2 provides the dose conversion from paliperidone palmitate to Invega Hafyera®, while Table 10.3 provides the dose conversion from Invega Trinza® to Invega Hafyera® [1].

M. J. Ehret, *Long-Acting Injectable Medications in Mental Health*, https://doi.org/10.1007/978-3-032-09415-5_10

Table 10.1 Dosing recommendations [1]

Initial dose	Based on previous paliperidone palmitate or Invega Trinza® dosing
Oral overlap	Not required
Target dose	Based on previous paliperidone palmitate or Invega Trinza® dosing
Maximum dose	1560 mg every 6 months
Dosing interval	Every 6 months
Renal/hepatic dosing	For patients with renal impairment (CrCl ≥50–<80 mL/min [Cockcroft-Gault Formula]), adjust dose and stabilize the patient using paliperidone palmitate before transitioning to Invega Hafyera® or from paliperidone palmitate to Invega Trinza® before transitioning to Invega Hafyera®. Not recommended in patients with moderate or severe renal impairment (CrCl <50 mL/min) No hepatic dosing noted in package insert

IM Intramuscular, *CrCl* Creatine clearance

Table 10.2 Dose conversion of paliperidone palmitate to Invega Hafyera® [1]

Last dose of Paliperidone Palmitate	Initial dose of Invega Hafyera®
156 mg	1092 mg
234 mg	1560 mg

Table 10.3 Dose Conversion of Invega Trinza® to Invega Hafyera® [1]

Last dose of Invega Trinza®	Initial dose of Invega Hafyera®
546 mg	1092 mg
819 mg	1560 mg

Table 10.4 Missed dose recommendations: more than 6 months and 3 weeks, up to less than 8 months since the last injection [1]

Last dose of Invega Hafyera®	Paliperidone Palmitate dose to be administered into the deltoid muscle	Invega Hafyera® dose to be administered into the gluteal muscle
	Day 1	1 month after day 1
1092 mg	156 mg	1092 mg
1560 mg	234 mg	1560 mg

- To avoid a missed dose, patients may be given the injection up to 2 weeks before or 3 weeks after the scheduled 6-month dose. Tables 10.4 and 10.5 provide details on how to manage missed doses of Invega Hafyera®.
- If more than 11 months have elapsed since the last dose of Invega Hafyera®, reinitiate with paliperidone palmitate as described in the prescribing information. Invega Hafyera® can then be resumed after the patient has been adequately treated with paliperidone palmitate for at least 4 months.

Table 10.5 Missed dose recommendations: 8 months up to and including 11 months since the last dose [1]

Last dose of Invega Hafyera®	Paliperidone Palmitate dose to be administered into the deltoid muscle		Invega Hafyera® dose to be administered into the gluteal muscle
	Day 1	Day 8	1 month after Day 8
1092 mg	156 mg	156 mg	1092 mg
1560 mg	156 mg	156 mg	1560 mg

Table 10.6 Pharmacokinetic properties [1, 2]

Half-life	Median apparent half-life ranges from 148 days to 159 days.
TMax	29–32 days
Therapeutic window	20–60 ng/mL.

TMax Time to maximum concentration

Pharmacokinetic Properties

Table 10.6 provides details on the pharmacokinetic properties [1, 2].

Drug Interactions

No specific drug interaction studies have been performed with Invega Hafyera® [1].

Adverse Reactions

Invega Hafyera® is generally well-tolerated with similar adverse effects as the oral paliperidone products. The most common adverse effects were agitation, akathisia, constipation, diarrhea, dizziness, headache, injection-site reactions, insomnia, nausea, somnolence, tachycardia, tremor, and weight gain [3].

Preparation and Administration Instructions

Invega Hafyera® is available as a prefilled syringe with 1092 and 1560 mg strengths. These syringes should be stored at room temperature. Table 10.7 provides details on the injection volume [1].

Injection site: Gluteal muscle

Administration instructions [1]:

Table 10.7 Injection volume [1]

Medication strength	Injection volume
1092 mg	3.5 mL
1560 mg	5 mL

- Must be administered as an intramuscular injection by a health-care professional. Do not administer by any other route.
- As a universal precaution, hands should be washed with soap and water prior to preparation and administration. Gloves should always be worn.
- Shake the prefilled syringe with the syringe tip-cap pointing upward very fast for at least 15 seconds, rest briefly, then shake again for 15 seconds. If more than 5 minutes pass before injection, shake the syringe very fast with the tip-cap pointing upward again for at least 30 seconds to resuspend Invega Hafyera®.
- Check the suspension for solid product. The suspension should appear uniform, thick, and milky white. It is normal to see air bubbles. If a solid product is seen, reshake the syringe with the syringe tip-cap pointing up very fast for at least 15 seconds, rest, then shake again for 15 seconds.
- Open the needle pouch.
- Remove the syringe tip cap and attach the needle with a gentle twisting motion to avoid needle hub cracks or damage.
- Pull back the plunger while holding the syringe upright.
- Gently pull back the plunger to clear the syringe tip of any solid product.
- Remove air bubbles by pressing the plunger carefully until a drop of liquid comes out of the needle tip.
- Remove the needle sheath from the needle in a straight motion.
- Use slow, firm, consistent pressure to press the plunger completely. This should take approximately 30 seconds. Continue to press the plunger if you feel resistance. This is normal.
- Dispose of the syringe in an appropriate sharps container.

References

1. Invega Hafyera® [package insert]. Titusville: Janssen Pharmaceuticals, Inc., 2025.
2. Schoretsanitis G, Bauman P, Conca A, et al. Therapeutic drug monitoring of long-acting injectable antipsychotic drugs. Ther Drug Monit. 2021;43:79–102.
3. Peters L, Dyer M, Schroeder E, et al. Invega Hafyera (paliperidone palmitate): extended-release injectable suspension for patients with schizophrenia. J Pharm Technol. 2023;39:88–94.

Chapter 11
Paliperidone Palmitate (Erzofri®): Second-Generation Antipsychotic Long-Acting Injectable

LAI Technology

Erzofri® uses a long-acting, extended-release delivery system.

Erzofri® is an atypical antipsychotic indicated for the treatment of schizophrenia in adults and the treatment of schizoaffective disorder in adults as monotherapy and as an adjunct to mood stabilizers or antidepressants [1].

Dosing Parameters

As with all long-acting injectables (LAIs), establishment of tolerability with prior oral administration is recommended prior to utilization of the LAI formulation. Table 11.1 provides dosing recommendations for Erzofri® [1].

Erzofri® has an established conversion of the oral formulation to the LAI formulation. Table 11.2 provides the dose conversion from oral paliperidone to Erzofri®.

When switching patients currently at steady state on another LAI, initiate Erzofri® in place of the next scheduled injection [1].

If an individual misses a scheduled injection of Erzofri®, an established missed dose schedule has been provided within the package insert. Table 11.3 provides clinical recommendations on how to manage missed doses of Erzofri® [1].

M. J. Ehret, *Long-Acting Injectable Medications in Mental Health*,
https://doi.org/10.1007/978-3-032-09415-5_11

Table 11.1 Dosing recommendations [1]

Initial dose	351 mg in the deltoid
Oral overlap	Not required
Target dose	117 mg
Maximum dose	234 mg
Dosing interval	Every 4 weeks
Renal/hepatic dosing	Mild renal impairment: CrCl >50–<80 mL/min (Cockcroft-Gault Formula), initiate Erzofri® with a dose of 234 mg on treatment day in the deltoid muscle. Follow with the recommended monthly maintenance dose of 78 mg, either deltoid or gluteal. The maximum dose is 156 mg. No hepatic dosing noted in package insert.

IM Intramuscular, *CrCl* Creatine clearance

Table 11.2 Dose conversion of oral to LAI [1]

Oral daily dose	LAI dose
3 mg paliperidone	39–78 mg Erzofri®
6 mg paliperidone	117 mg Erzofri®
9 mg paliperidone	156 mg Erzofri®
12 mg paliperidone	234 mg Erzofri®

LAI Long-acting injectable antipsychotic medication

Table 11.3 Missed dose recommendations [1]

Timing of missed dose	How to manage
4–6 weeks	Resume regular monthly dosing as soon as possible
>6 weeks–6 months	Resume the same dose the patient was previously stabilized on (unless the patient was stabilized on a dose of 234 mg, then the first 2 injections should each be 156 mg): Administer a deltoid injection as soon as possible Administer a second deltoid injection 1 week later at the same dose Resume administering the previously stabilized dose in the deltoid or gluteal muscle 1 month after the second injection
>6 months	Restart with the recommended initiation: Administer a 351 mg deltoid injection on Day 1 Thereafter, resume administering the previously stabilized dose in the deltoid or gluteal 1 month after the initial injection.

Table 11.4 Pharmacokinetic properties

Half-life	27 days
TMax	16–28 days
Therapeutic window	20–60 ng/mL

TMax Time to maximum concentration

Pharmacokinetic Properties

Table 11.4 provides the pharmacokinetic properties of Erzofri® [1, 2].

Drug Interactions

Erzofri® should be avoided with a strong inducer of CYP3A4 and/or p-glycoprotein medications during the 1-month dosing interval for Erzofri®, if possible. If administering a strong inducer is necessary, consider managing the patient using paliperidone extended-release tablets [1].

Adverse Reactions

Erzofri® is generally well tolerated with similar adverse effects as the oral paliperidone products. The most common adverse effects were agitation, akathisia, constipation, diarrhea, dizziness, headache, injection-site reactions, insomnia, nausea, somnolence, tachycardia, tremor, and weight gain [1].

Preparation and Administration Instructions

Erzofri® is available as a prefilled syringe with 39, 78, 117, 156, 234, and 351 mg strengths. These syringes should be stored at room temperature. Table 11.5 provides the injection volumes [1].

Injection site: Deltoid muscle on Day 1; subsequent dosages may be administered in the deltoid or gluteal muscle.

Administration instructions [1]:

- Must be administered as an intramuscular injection by a health-care professional. Do not administer by any other route.
- As a universal precaution, hands should be washed with soap and water prior to preparation and administration. Gloves should always be worn.
- Shake the syringe vigorously for a minimum of 10 seconds to ensure a homogeneous suspension.

Table 11.5 Injection volume [1]

Medication strength	Injection volume
39 mg	0.25 mL
78 mg	0.5 mL
117 mg	0.75 mL
156 mg	1 mL
234 mg	1.5 mL
351 mg	2.25 mL

Table 11.6 Needle size selection [1]

Injection site	Needle size
Deltoid	Patients weighing <90 kg: 1 inch (23G) Patients weighing >90 kg: 1.5 inch (22G)
Gluteal	1.5 inch (22G)

- Select the appropriate needle and injection site. Table 11.6 provides the needle size for the injection sites.
- Hold the syringe with the tip-cap pointing upward. Remove the rubber tip with an easy counterclockwise twisting motion.
- Peel the safety needle pouch halfway open. Grasp the needle sheath using the plastic peel pouch. Hold the syringe pointing upward. Attach the safety needle to the syringe using a gentle twisting motion to avoid needle hub cracks or damage.
- Pull the needle sheath away from the needle with a straight pull.
- Bring the syringe with the attached needle in an upright position to deaerate. Deaerate the syringe by moving the plunger rod carefully forward.
- Inject the entire contents intramuscularly slowly, deep into the selected deltoid or gluteal muscle.
- Dispose of the syringe in an appropriate sharps container.

References

1. Erzofri® [package insert]. Yantai: Shandong Luye Pharmaceutical Co., Ltd.; 2025.
2. Scoretsanitis G, Bauman P, Conca A, et al. Therapeutic drug monitoring of long-acting injectable antipsychotic drugs. Ther Drug Monit. 2021;43:79–102.

Chapter 12
Risperidone Long-Acting Injection (Risperdal Consta®): Second-Generation Antipsychotic Long-Acting Injectable

LAI Technology

Risperdal Consta® is manufactured using a novel drug delivery system in which the active medication, risperidone, is encapsulated in a Medisorb polymer to form microspheres. The polymer contains the metabolic precursors of two naturally occurring compounds, lactic acid and glycolic acid. They are linked together to form chains of varying lengths. At the time of administration, the microspheres are suspended in an aqueous diluent and then hydrolyzed to gradually release the medication. The end byproducts of the breakdown of the microspheres are carbon dioxide and water [1]. The release of the risperidone takes at least 3 weeks.

Risperdal Consta® is an atypical antipsychotic indicated for the treatment of schizophrenia and as monotherapy or as adjunctive therapy to lithium or valproate for the maintenance treatment of bipolar I disorder [2].

Dosing Parameters

As with all long-acting injectables (LAIs), establishment of tolerability with prior oral administration is recommended prior to utilization of the LAI formulation. Table 12.1 provides the dosing recommendations for Risperdal Consta® [2].

Risperdal Consta® has an established conversion of the oral formulation to the LAI formulation. Table 12.2 provides the dose conversion of oral risperidone to Risperdal Consta®.

If an individual should miss a scheduled injection of Risperdal Consta®, an established missed dose schedule has been recommended in the literature. Table 12.3 describes how to manage a missed dose [4].

M. J. Ehret, *Long-Acting Injectable Medications in Mental Health*,
https://doi.org/10.1007/978-3-032-09415-5_12

Table 12.1 Dosing recommendations [2]

Initial dose	25 mg IM
Oral overlap	21 days
Target dose	25–50 mg
Maximum dose	50 mg
Dosing interval	Every 2 weeks
Renal/hepatic dosing	12.5 mg may be substituted for the 25 mg dose when clinically appropriate (i.e., hepatic and/or renal impairment, drug interactions which may increase risperidone plasma concentrations, or history of medication intolerance)

IM Intramuscular

Table 12.2 Dose conversion of oral to LAI [2, 3]

Oral daily dose of Risperidone	LAI dose[a]
1 mg	12.5 mg Risperdal Consta®
2–3 mg	25 mg Risperdal Consta®
3–5 mg	37.5 mg Risperdal Consta®
4–5 mg	50 mg Risperdal Consta®

LAI Long-acting injectable antipsychotic medication
[a]Do not combine different dosage strengths in a single administration

Table 12.3 Missed dose recommendations [4]

Time since last injection	How to manage
Patient is not at steady state and >2 weeks since the last dose	Give the next injection as soon as possible, plus oral supplementation for 3 weeks
Patient at steady state and <6weeks since the last injection	Give the next injection as soon as possible
Patient at steady state and >6 weeks since the last injection	Give the next injection as soon as possible, plus oral supplementation for 3 weeks

Table 12.4 Pharmacokinetic properties [5]

Half-life	3–6 days
TMax	21 days (main release begins)
Time to steady state	After the fourth injection
Therapeutic window	20–60 ng/mL

Information from: Schorestsanitis [5]
TMax Time to maximum concentration

Pharmacokinetic Properties

After a single dose of the injection, there is a small release of the medication (<1%), followed by a lag time of approximately 3 weeks. Following continuous exposure to body water for 3 weeks, the main release of the medication begins as the microspheres break down. Seven weeks after the intramuscular injection, the release of the medication discontinues [1]. Table 12.4 provides the pharmacokinetic properties [5].

Drug Interactions

Risperdal Consta® coadministration with CYP3A4 enzyme inducers would be expected to cause decreases in the plasma concentrations of the sum of risperidone and 9-hydroxyrisperidone combined, which could lead to decreased efficacy of Risperdal Consta® treatment. The dose of risperidone needs to be titrated for patients receiving these enzyme inducers, especially during initiation or discontinuation of therapy with these inducers. At the initiation of a CYP3A4 inducer medication, patients should be closely monitored during the first 4–8 weeks, since the dose of Risperdal Consta® may need to be adjusted. A dose increase, or additional oral risperidone, may be considered. On discontinuation of CYP3A4 inducers, the dosage of Risperdal Consta® should be reevaluated and, if necessary, decreased. Patients may need to be placed on a lower dose of Risperdal Consta® between 2 and 4 weeks before the planned discontinuation of CYP3A4 inducer medications to adjust for the expected increase in plasma concentrations of risperidone plus 9-hydroxyrisperidone. For patients treated with the recommended dose of 25 mg of Risperdal Consta® and discontinuing CYP3A4 inducer medications, it is recommended to continue treatment with the 25 mg dose unless clinical judgment necessitates lowering the Risperdal Consta® dose to 12.5 mg or necessitates interruption of Risperdal Consta® treatment [6].

Medications that inhibit CYP2D6 have been shown to increase the plasma concentration of risperidone. When either concomitant fluoxetine or paroxetine is initiated or discontinued, reevaluation of the dose of Risperdal Consta® should be completed. When initiation of fluoxetine or paroxetine is considered, patients may be placed on a lower dose of Risperdal Consta® between 2 and 4 weeks before the planned start of fluoxetine or paroxetine therapy to adjust for the expected increase in plasma concentrations of risperidone. When fluoxetine or paroxetine is initiated in patients receiving the recommended dose of 25 mg Risperdal Consta®, it is recommended to continue treatment with the 25 mg dose unless clinical judgment necessitates lowering the Risperdal Consta® dose to 12.5 mg or necessitates interruption of Risperdal Consta® treatment. When Risperdal Consta® is initiated in patients already receiving fluoxetine or paroxetine, a starting dose of 12.5 mg can be considered [6].

Adverse Reactions

Beyond pain at the injection site, the adverse effects from Risperdal Consta® are similar to those of oral risperidone. The most common adverse effects include akathisia, dizziness, headache, insomnia, Parkinsonism, and somnolence [2].

Preparation and Administration Instructions

Risperdal Consta® is available as a kit requiring reconstitution per the instructions detailed below. The entire dose pack should be stored in the refrigerator (2–8 °C/36°–46 °F) and protected from light. If refrigeration is unavailable, Risperdal Consta® can be stored at temperatures not exceeding 77 °F (25 °C) for no more than 7 days prior to administration [2].

Injection site: Gluteal (upper-outer quadrant) or deltoid muscle

Injection volume: 2 mL

Administration instructions [2]:

- Must be administered as an intramuscular injection by a health-care professional. Do not administer by any other route.
- As a universal precaution, hands should be washed with soap and water prior to preparation and administration. Gloves should always be worn.
- May be used up to 6 hours after suspension (store at room temperature); resuspend, if necessary, before administering.
- The Risperdal Consta® kit needs to be removed from the refrigerator 30 minutes prior to reconstituting. It should not be warmed up any other way.
- The cap should be removed from the vial and wiped with an alcohol swab.
- Holding the sterile blister, the back of the vial adapter should be peeled back and removed.
- The vial adapter should be pushed onto the vial top until it snaps securely into place.
- Remove the sterile blister.
- Hold the white collar at the tip of the syringe and remove the cap.
- Connect the syringe to the vial adapter using a clockwise twisting motion until it feels snug.
- Inject the diluent from the syringe into the vial.
- Shake vigorously for at least 10 seconds. Check the suspension to verify it is uniform, thick, and milky in color. Microspheres will be visible in the liquid.
- Invert the vial and slowly pull the plunger rod to withdraw the entire contents from the vial to the syringe.
- Hold the white collar on the syringe and unscrew the vial adapter.
- Tear a section of the vial label at the perforation. Apply the detached label to the syringe for identification purposes.
- Select the appropriate needle and injection site. Table 12.5 provides the needle size for the injection sites.
- Attach the needle with a clockwise twisting motion until snug.
- Resuspend the microspheres by shaking vigorously, as some settling will occur.
- Pull the needle sheath off in a straight motion.

Table 12.5 Needle size selection [2]

Injection site	Needle size
Deltoid	1 inch (21G)
Gluteal	2 inches (20G)

- Hold the needle upright and tap gently to make any air bubbles rise to the top. Slowly and carefully press the plunger rod upward to remove the air.
- Immediately inject the entire contents of the syringe intramuscularly into the gluteal or deltoid muscle of the patient.
- Dispose of the syringe in an appropriate sharps container.

References

1. Ehret MJ, Fuller MA. Long-acting injectable risperidone. Ann Pharmacother. 2004;38:2122–7.
2. Risperdal Consta® [package insert]. Titusville: Janssen Pharmaceuticals, Inc.; 2025.
3. Bai YM, Chen TT, Chen JY, et al. Equivalent switching dose from oral risperidone to risperidone long-acting injection: a 48-week randomized, prospective, single-blind pharmacokinetic study. J Clin Psychiatry. 2007;8:1218–25.
4. Carpenter J, Wong KK. Use a stepwise approach based on the unique properties of the specific medication. Curr Psychiatr Ther. 2018;17:11–20.
5. Schoretsanitis G, Bauman P, Conca A, et al. Therapeutic drug monitoring of long-acting injectable antipsychotic drugs. Ther Drug Monit. 2021;43:79–102.
6. Stahl SM. The prescriber's guide: Stahl's essential psychopharmacology. 6th ed. New York: Cambridge University Press; 2017.

Chapter 13
Risperidone for Extended-Release Injectable Suspension (Perseris®): Second-Generation Antipsychotic Long-Acting Injectable

LAI Technology

Perseris® uses an Atrigel® system, which consists of biodegradable polymers dissolved in a liquid. After injection, it solidifies upon contact with aqueous body fluids to form a solid implant. The implant then delivers risperidone in a controlled fashion over an extended period of time. Appropriate administration technique, as a subcutaneous injection, is essential to avoid injection into a vein or muscle due to the technology [1].

Perseris® is an atypical antipsychotic indicated for the treatment of schizophrenia in adults.

Dosing Parameters

As with all long-acting injectables (LAIs), establishment of tolerability with prior oral administration is recommended prior to utilization of the LAI formulation. Table 13.1 provides details on the dosing recommendations for Perseris® [1].

Perseris® has an established conversion of the oral formulation to the LAI formulation. Table 13.2 provides the dose conversion of oral risperidone to Perseris®.

If an individual should miss a scheduled injection of Perseris®, the next injection should be administered as soon as possible.

M. J. Ehret, *Long-Acting Injectable Medications in Mental Health*,
https://doi.org/10.1007/978-3-032-09415-5_13

Table 13.1 Dosing recommendations [1]

Initial dose	Based on the oral risperidone dose
Oral overlap	Not required
Target dose	Based on the oral risperidone dose
Maximum dose	120 mg every 4 weeks
Dosing interval	Every 4 weeks
Renal/hepatic dosing	Titrate with oral risperidone up to at least 3 mg daily. Following oral titration and based on clinical response and tolerability, the recommended dose of Perseris® is 90 mg once monthly.

Table 13.2 Dose conversion of oral to LAI [1]

Oral daily dose	LAI dose
3 mg risperidone	90 mg 1 day after the last oral risperidone dose
4 mg risperidone	120 mg 1 day after the last oral risperidone dose

LAI Long-acting injectable antipsychotic medication

Table 13.3 Pharmacokinetic Properties [1, 2]

Half-life	8–11 days
TMax	4–6 hours (first peak) 10–14 days (second peak)
Time to steady state	After two injections
Therapeutic window	20–60 ng/mL

TMax Time to maximum concentration

Pharmacokinetic Properties

After a single subcutaneous injection, there is a rapid absorption of risperidone with an initial peak at 4 hours. Over the next 11 days, there is a slow increase in the combined levels of risperidone and 9-hydroxyrisperidone until the peak is reached. Table 13.3 provides the pharmacokinetic properties [1, 2].

Drug Interactions

Between 2 and 4 weeks prior to initiating a strong CYP2D6 inhibitor, switch patients to the lowest Perseris® dosage (90 mg once monthly) to adjust for the expected increase in plasma concentrations of risperidone [1].

With concomitant use of Perseris® 90 mg and strong CYP3A4 inducers, increase Perseris® dosage to 120 mg once monthly and consider starting additional oral risperidone therapy. In patients already receiving Perseris® 120 mg once monthly, additional oral risperidone therapy may be considered [1].

Upon discontinuation of a strong CYP3A4 inducer in patients receiving Perseris® 120 mg once monthly, reevaluate the dosage of Perseris® or any additional oral risperidone therapy and, if necessary, decrease to adjust for the expected increase in plasma concentrations of risperidone [1].

Upon discontinuation of a strong CYP3A4 inducer in a patient receiving Perseris® 90 mg once monthly, continue treatment with the 90 mg dose unless clinical judgment necessitates interruption of Perseris® treatment [1].

Adverse Reactions

Beyond pain at the injection site, the adverse effects from Perseris® are similar to those of oral risperidone. The most common adverse effects include akathisia, dizziness, headache, insomnia, Parkinsonism, and somnolence [1].

Preparation and Administration Instructions

Perseris® is available as a single-dose kit of 90 and 120 mg strengths requiring reconstitution per the instructions detailed below. The entire pack should be stored in the refrigerator at 2–8 °C (36–46 °F). Perseris® may be stored unopened original packaging at room temperature, 20–25 °C (68–77 °F), for up to 30 days. After removal from the refrigerator, use Perseris® within 30 days or discard. Table 13.4 provides the injection volume [1].

Injection site: Subcutaneous injection in the abdomen or the back of the upper arm

Administration instructions [1]:

- Must be administered as a subcutaneous injection by a health-care professional. Do not administer by any other route.
- As a universal precaution, hands should be washed with soap and water prior to preparation and administration. Gloves should always be worn.
- Allow Perseris® kit to come to room temperature for at least 15 minutes prior to mixing.
- Hold the powder syringe upright and tap the barrel of the syringe to dislodge the packed powder.
- Remove the cap from the liquid syringe, then remove the cap from the powder syringe.

Table 13.4 Injection volume [1]

Mediation strength	Injection volume
90 mg	0.6 mL
120 mg	0.8 mL

- Place the liquid syringe on top of the powder syringe and connect the syringes by twisting approximately ¾ turn. Keep your fingers off the plungers during this step to avoid spillage of the medication.
- Transfer the contents of the liquid syringe into the powder syringe.
- Gently push the powder syringe plunger until you feel resistance.
- Repeat this gentle back-and-forth process for five cycles (one cycle is a back-and-forth between the two syringes).
- Continue mixing the syringes for an additional 55 cycles.
- This mixing can be more vigorous than the first five cycles.
- Transfer all contents into the liquid syringe.
- Maintain slight pressure on the powder syringe plunger and pull back gently on the liquid syringe plunger while twisting the syringes apart.
- Attach the safety needle by twisting it.
- Check that the medication is uniform in color and free from foreign particles.
- Clean the skin with an alcohol pad.
- Hold the syringe upright for several seconds to allow air bubbles to rise. Remove the needle sheath and slowly depress the plunger to push out the excess air from the syringe.
- Pinch the skin around the injection area. Insert the needle fully into the subcutaneous tissue and inject the medication slowly and steadily.
- Withdraw the needle at the same angle used for insertion and release pinched skin. Do not rub the injection area after the injection.
- Dispose of the syringe in an appropriate sharps container.

References

1. Perseris® [package insert]. North Chesterfield: Indivior, Inc.; 2025.
2. Schoretsanitis G, Bauman P, Conca A, et al. Therapeutic drug monitoring of long-acting injectable antipsychotic drugs. Ther Drug Monit. 2021;43:79–102.

Chapter 14
Risperidone Extended-Release Injectable Suspension (Uzedy®): Second-Generation Antipsychotic Long-Acting Injectable

LAI Technology

Uzedy® utilizes SteadyTeq™, a copolymer technology, which is proprietary to MedinCell. It controls the rate and duration of risperidone release. With this delivery system, therapeutic blood concentrations are reached within the first 6–24 hours after a single injection [1, 2].

Uzedy® is an atypical antipsychotic indicated for the treatment of schizophrenia in adults and as monotherapy or as adjunctive therapy to lithium or valproate for the maintenance treatment of bipolar I disorder in adults [2].

Dosing Parameters

As with all long-acting injectables (LAIs), establishment of tolerability with prior oral administration is recommended prior to utilization of the LAI formulation. Table 14.1 provides details on the dosing recommendations for Uzedy® [2].

Uzedy® has an established conversion of the oral formulation to the LAI formulation. Table 14.2 provides the dose conversion from oral risperidone to either the monthly or every 2-month formulations of Uzedy® [2].

Patients can switch between monthly and every 2 months by administering the first dose of the new dosing regimen on the next scheduled date of administration in the original dosing regimen [2].

M. J. Ehret, *Long-Acting Injectable Medications in Mental Health*,
https://doi.org/10.1007/978-3-032-09415-5_14

Table 14.1 Dosing recommendations [2]

Initial dose	Based on the dose of oral risperidone
Oral overlap	Not required
Target dose	Based on the dose of oral risperidone
Maximum dose	125 mg every 4 weeks or 250 mg every 8 weeks
Dosing interval	Every 4 or 8 weeks
Renal/hepatic dosing	Titrate with oral risperidone to at least 2 mg once daily. Following oral titration, and based on clinical response and tolerability, the recommended dose of Uzedy® is 50 mg once a month.

Table 14.2 Dose conversion of oral to LAI [2]

Oral daily dose	LAI dose once monthly	LAI dose every 8 weeks
2 mg risperidone	50 mg	100 mg
3 mg risperidone	75 mg	150 mg
4 mg risperidone	100 mg	200 mg
5 mg risperidone	125 mg	250 mg

LAI Long-acting injectable antipsychotic medication

Table 14.3 Pharmacokinetic properties [2, 3]

Half-life	Mean apparent half-life ranges between 14 days and 22 days
TMax	8–14 days
Time to steady state	2 months
Therapeutic window	20–60 ng/mL

TMax Time to maximum concentration

If an individual misses a scheduled injection of Uzedy®, the next injection should be administered as soon as possible. Do not administer it more frequently than recommended [2].

Pharmacokinetic Properties

Table 14.3 provides pharmacokinetic properties [2, 3].

Drug Interactions

When initiation of fluoxetine or paroxetine is considered, place patients on a lower dose of Uzedy® prior to the planned start of fluoxetine or paroxetine therapy to adjust for the expected increase in plasma concentrations of risperidone. When fluoxetine or paroxetine is initiated in patients receiving the recommended dose of

50 mg once monthly or 100 mg once every 2 months of Uzedy®, continue treatment with these doses unless clinical judgment necessitates interruption of Uzedy® [2].

At the initiation of therapy with strong CYP3A4 inducers, patients should be closely monitored during the first 4–8 weeks since the dose of Uzedy® may need to be adjusted. A dose increase, or additional oral risperidone, may be considered. On discontinuation of a strong CYP3A4 inducer, reevaluate the dosage of Uzedy® or any additional oral risperidone therapy and, if necessary, adjust for the expected increase in plasma concentration of risperidone. On discontinuation of a strong CYP3A4 inducer in a patient treated with Uzedy® 50 mg once monthly or 100 mg once every 2 months, continue treatment with these doses unless clinical judgment necessitates interruption of Uzedy® [2].

Adverse Reactions

Beyond pain at the injection site, the adverse effects from Uzedy® are similar to those of oral risperidone. The most common adverse effects include akathisia, dizziness, headache, insomnia, Parkinsonism, and somnolence [2].

Preparation and Administration Instructions

Uzedy® is a prefilled syringe available in 50, 75, 100, 125, 150, 200, and 250 mg strengths. It should be stored in the refrigerator at 2–8 °C (36–46 °F) in the original carton to protect it from light. Uzedy® may be stored unopened original packaging at room temperature, 20–25 °C (68–77 °F), for up to 90 days. If unopened, Uzedy® may be returned to refrigerated storage within 90 days. Once the carton is opened, administer Uzedy® or discard. Table 14.4 provides injection volumes for the various strengths [2].

Injection site: Abdominal or upper arm subcutaneous injection

Administration instructions [2]:

- Must be administered as a subcutaneous injection by a health-care professional. Do not administer by any other route.

Table 14.4 Injection volume [2]

Injection strength	Injection volume
50 mg	0.14 mL
75 mg	0.21 mL
100 mg	0.28 mL
125 mg	0.35 mL
150 mg	0.42 mL
200 mg	0.56 mL
250 mg	0.7 mL

- As a universal precaution, hands should be washed with soap and water prior to preparation and administration. Gloves should always be worn.
- Remove the kit from the refrigerator and allow it to sit at room temperature for at least 30 minutes. Uzedy® is a solid at refrigerated temperatures and must reach room temperature prior to administration. Do not warm it by any other method, and keep it protected from light.
- Verify the medication is white to off-white, opaque in color, and free from non-white particulate matter.
- Expose the safety needle hub by peeling back the paper tab of the needle pouch.
- Firmly hold the syringe with the white collar and flick the syringe forcefully three times to move the bubble to the cap. Failure to move the bubble to the cap of the syringe could result in incomplete dosage. The flick of the syringe is like a whip of the syringe.
- Check that the bubble is at the cap of the syringe. If the bubble is not at the cap, repeat flicking/whipping until the bubble is at the top of the syringe.
- Hold the syringe vertically with the white collar and bend and snap off the cap.
- Hold the syringe vertically with the white collar at the top and push the green hub of the safety needle inside the white collar of the syringe. Rotate the safety needle while holding the white collar until it is secure and tight.
- Select the injection site and clean with an alcohol pad.
- Remove the needle sheath by pulling it away from the green hub. Do not expel any visible air bubbles.
- Pinch at least 1 inch of the area of cleaned skin with your free hand.
- Insert the needle into the subcutaneous tissue. Release the pinched skin once the needle is in the subcutaneous tissue.
- Push on the plunger using a slow, firm, and steady push until the entire dose is delivered. Inject the entire dose at one time.
- Resistance will be experienced during dose delivery.
- Wait 2–3 seconds after the entire dose is delivered before removing the needle. Slowly pull the needle out from the injection site at the same angle as insertion.
- Dispose of the syringe in an appropriate sharps container.

References

1. Kane J, Haray E, et al. Efficacy and safety of TV-46000, a long-acting, subcutaneous, injectable formulation of risperidone, for schizophrenia: a randomized clinical trial in the USA and Bulgaria. Lancet Psychiatry. 2023;10:935–44.
2. Uzedy® [package insert]. Parsippany: Teva Neuroscience, Inc.; 2025.
3. Schoretsanitis G, Bauman P, Conca A, et al. Therapeutic drug monitoring of long-acting injectable antipsychotic drugs. Ther Drug Monit. 2021;43:79–102.

Chapter 15
Risperidone for Extended-Release Injectable Suspension (Rykindo®): Second-Generation Antipsychotic Long-Acting Injectable

LAI Technology

Rykindo® is an innovative microsphere formulation that has been independently developed by Luye Pharmaceuticals. Rykindo® is delivered via long-acting injectable (LAI) and extended-release microsphere technology. The microspheres are released at a gradual, steady rate [1].

Rykindo® is an atypical antipsychotic indicated for the treatment of schizophrenia in adults and as monotherapy or as adjunctive therapy to lithium or valproate for the maintenance treatment of bipolar I disorder in adults [1].

Dosing Parameters

As with all LAIs, establishment of tolerability with prior oral administration is recommended prior to utilization of the LAI formulation. Table 15.1 provides the dosing recommendations for Rykindo® [1].

Rykindo® does not have an established conversion of the oral formulation to the LAI formulation. The following dose conversion is based on clinical expertise. Table 15.2 provides the dose conversion of oral risperidone to Rykindo® [1].

Patients who receive risperidone long-acting injection 2-week IM formulation (e.g., Risperdal Consta®), the Rykindo® dose should be the same as that of previous treatment with Risperdal Consta®. The first injection of Rykindo® should be given 4 weeks (no later than 5 weeks) after the last injection of the previous treatment. Supplementation with oral risperidone is not recommended. Titration should not be done more frequently than every 4 weeks [1].

When restarting patients who have had an interval of treatment with Rykindo®, the previously established dosage should be reinitiated if there has been no change

M. J. Ehret, *Long-Acting Injectable Medications in Mental Health*,
https://doi.org/10.1007/978-3-032-09415-5_15

Table 15.1 Dosing recommendations [1]

Initial dose	25 mg
Oral overlap	7 days of oral risperidone
Target dose	25 mg
Maximum dose	50 mg
Dosing interval	Every 2 weeks
Renal/hepatic dosing	Titrate with oral risperidone up to at least 2 mg before initiating treatment with Rykindo®. A starting dose of 12.5 mg may be appropriate for some patients.

IM Intramuscular

Table 15.2 Dose conversion of oral to LAI [1]

Oral daily dose of risperidone	LAI dose[a]
1 mg	12.5 mg Rykindo®
2–3 mg	25 mg Rykindo®
3–5 mg	37.5 mg Rykindo®
4–5 mg	50 mg Rykindo®

LAI Long-acting injectable antipsychotic medication
[a]Do not combine different dosage strengths in a single administration

Table 15.3 Pharmacokinetic properties [1, 2]

Half-life	Apparent half-life is 3–6 days
TMax	14–17 days
Therapeutic window	20–60 ng/mL

TMax Time to maximum concentration

in the patient's general medical condition. Supplementation with oral risperidone is also required [1].

Pharmacokinetic Properties

Table 15.3 provides pharmacokinetic properties [1, 2].

Drug Interactions

Rykindo® coadministration with CYP3A4 enzyme inducers would be expected to cause decreases in the plasma concentrations of the sum of risperidone and 9-hydroxyrisperidone combined, which could lead to decreased efficacy of Rykindo® treatment. The dose of risperidone needs to be titrated for patients receiving these enzyme inducers, especially during initiation or discontinuation of therapy with these inducers. At the initiation of a CYP3A4 inducer medication, patients should be closely monitored during the first 4–8 weeks, since the dose of Rykindo® may need to be adjusted. A dose increase, or additional oral risperidone, may be considered. On discontinuation of CYP3A4 inducers, the dosage of Rykindo® should be reevaluated and, if necessary, decreased. Patients may need to be placed on a lower dose of Rykindo® between 2 and 4 weeks before the planned discontinuation of CYP3A4 inducer medications to adjust for the expected increase in plasma concentrations of risperidone plus 9-hydroxyrisperidone. For patients treated with the recommended dose of 25 mg of Rykindo® and discontinuing CYP3A4 inducer medications, it is recommended to continue treatment with the 25-mg dose unless clinical judgment necessitates lowering the Rykindo® dose to 12.5 mg or necessitates interruption of Rykindo® treatment [1].

Medications that inhibit CYP2D6 have been shown to increase the plasma concentration of risperidone. When either concomitant fluoxetine or paroxetine is initiated or discontinued, reevaluation of the dose of Risperdal Consta® should be completed. When initiation of fluoxetine or paroxetine is considered, patients may be placed on a lower dose of Rykindo® between 2 and 4 weeks before the planned start of fluoxetine or paroxetine therapy to adjust for the expected increase in plasma concentrations of risperidone. When fluoxetine or paroxetine is initiated in patients receiving the recommended dose of 25 mg Rykindo®, it is recommended to continue treatment with the 25 mg dose unless clinical judgment necessitates lowering the Rykindo® dose to 12.5 mg or necessitates interruption of Risperdal Consta® treatment. When Rykindo® is initiated in patients already receiving fluoxetine or paroxetine, a starting dose of 12.5 mg can be considered [1].

Adverse Reactions

Beyond pain at the injection site, the adverse effects from Rykindo® are similar to those of oral risperidone. The most common adverse effects include akathisia, dizziness, headache, insomnia, Parkinsonism, and somnolence [1].

Preparation and Administration Instructions

Rykindo® is available as a kit requiring reconstitution per the instructions detailed below. The entire dose pack should be stored in the refrigerator (2–8 °C/36–46 °F) and protected from light. If refrigeration is unavailable, Rykindo® can be stored at temperatures not exceeding 77 °F (25 °C) for no more than 7 days before administration. After removal from the refrigerator, use Rykindo® within 7 days or discard [1].

Injection site: Gluteal muscle

Injection Volume: 2 mL

Administration instructions [1]:

- Must be administered as an intramuscular injection by a health-care professional. Do not administer by any other route.
- As a universal precaution, hands should be washed with soap and water prior to preparation and administration. Gloves should always be worn.
- The Rykindo® kit needs to be removed from the refrigerator 30 minutes before reconstituting. It should not be warmed up any other way.
- The cap should be removed from the vial and wiped with an alcohol swab.
- Holding the sterile blister, the back of the vial adapter should be peeled back and removed.
- The vial adapter should be pushed onto the vial top until it snaps securely into place.
- Remove the sterile blister.
- Hold the luer-lock adapter at the tip of the syringe. Unscrew the translucent gray cap.
- Connect the syringe to the luer-lock adapter using a clockwise twisting motion until it feels snug.
- Inject the diluent from the syringe into the vial.
- Shake vigorously for at least 30 seconds. Check the suspension to verify it is uniform, thick, and milky in color.
- Invert the vial and slowly pull the plunger rod to withdraw the entire contents from the vial to the syringe.
- Hold the luer-lock adapter on the syringe and unscrew the vial adapter.
- Tear a section of the vial label at the perforation. Apply the detached label to the syringe for identification purposes.
- Take the needle out for a gluteal injection.
- Attach the needle with a clockwise twisting motion until snug.
- Resuspend the microspheres by shaking vigorously for 20–30 seconds, as some settling will occur.
- Pull the needle sheath off in a straight motion.
- Hold the needle upright and tap gently to make any air bubbles rise to the top. Slowly and carefully press the plunger rod upward to remove the air.
- Immediately inject the entire contents of the syringe intramuscularly into the gluteal muscle of the patient.
- Dispose of the syringe in an appropriate sharps container.

References

1. Rykindo® [package insert]. Yantai: Shandong Luye Pharmaceutical Co., Ltd; 2023.
2. Schoretsanitis G, Bauman P, Conca A, et al. Therapeutic drug monitoring of long-acting injectable antipsychotic drugs. Ther Drug Monit. 2021;43:79–102.

Chapter 16
Risperidone for Extended-Release Injectable Suspension (Risvan®): Second-Generation Antipsychotic Long-Acting Injectable

LAI Technology

Risvan® uses an ISM® technology platform, which is based on the in-situ formation of biodegradable matrices after the administration of a liquid carrier. It allows for therapeutic levels to be obtained quickly after administration [1].

Risvan® is an atypical antipsychotic indicated for the treatment of schizophrenia in adults [1].

Dosing Parameters

As with all long-acting injectables (LAIs), establishment of tolerability with prior oral administration is recommended before utilization of the LAI formulation. Table 16.1 provides the dosing recommendation for Risvan® [1].

Risvan® has an established conversion of the oral formulation to the LAI formulation. Table 16.2 provides the dose conversion of oral risperidone to Risvan®.

If an individual should miss a scheduled injection of Risvan®, the next dose should be administered as soon as possible. Do not administer more than one Risvan® dose per month.

M. J. Ehret, *Long-Acting Injectable Medications in Mental Health*, https://doi.org/10.1007/978-3-032-09415-5_16

Table 16.1 Dosing recommendations [1]

Initial dose	Based on the oral risperidone dose
Oral overlap	Not required
Target dose	Based on the oral risperidone dose
Maximum dose	100 mg once monthly
Dosing interval	Every 4 weeks
Renal/hepatic dosing	Titrate with oral risperidone to at least 3 mg before initiating treatment with Risvan®. Following oral titration, the recommended dosage of Risvan® is 75 mg once a month.

IM Intramuscular

Table 16.2 Dose conversion of oral to LAI [1]

Oral daily dose	LAI dose
3 mg risperidone	75 mg Risvan® dose 1 day after the last oral risperidone dose
4 mg risperidone	100 mg Risvan® dose 1 day after the last oral risperidone dose

LAI Long-acting injectable antipsychotic medication

Table 16.3 Pharmacokinetic properties [1, 2]

Half-life	3.9–7.5 days
TMax	Initial peak: 24–48 hours Second peak: Day 18–25
Therapeutic window	20–60 ng/mL

TMax Time to maximum concentration

Pharmacokinetic Properties

Table 16.3 provides pharmacokinetic properties [1, 2].

Drug Interactions

Between 2 and 4 weeks before initiating a strong CYP2D6 inhibitor, switch patients to the lowest Risvan® dosage (75 mg once monthly) to adjust for the expected increase in plasma concentrations of risperidone [1]. When a strong CYP2D6 inhibitor is initiated in patients receiving Risvan® 75 mg, continue treatment with 75 mg unless clinical judgment necessitates interruption of Risvan® treatment [1].

With concomitant use of Risvan® 75 mg and strong CYP3A4 inducers, increase Risvan® dosage to 100 mg once monthly. In patients already receiving Risvan® 100 mg once monthly, additional oral risperidone therapy may be considered [1].

Upon discontinuation of a strong CYP3A4 inducer in patients receiving Risvan® 100 mg once monthly, reevaluate the dosage of Risvan® or any additional oral risperidone therapy and, if necessary, decrease to adjust for the expected increase in plasma concentrations of risperidone [1].

Upon discontinuation of a strong CYP3A4 inducer in a patient receiving Risvan® 75 mg once monthly, continue treatment with the 75 mg dose unless clinical judgment necessitates interruption of Risvan® treatment [1].

Adverse Reactions

Beyond pain at the injection site, the adverse effects from Risvan® are similar to those of oral risperidone. The most common adverse effects include akathisia, dizziness, headache, insomnia, Parkinsonism, and somnolence [1].

Preparation and Administration Instructions

Risvan® is available as a single-dose kit of 75 and 100 mg strengths requiring reconstitution per the instructions detailed below. The entire pack should be stored at room temperature [1].

Injection site: Deltoid or gluteal muscle

Injection volume: Information not available

Administration instructions [1]:

- Must be administered as an intramuscular injection by a health-care professional. Do not administer by any other route.
- As a universal precaution, hands should be washed with soap and water prior to preparation and administration. Gloves should always be worn.
- Ensure the liquid syringe content flows normally. If frozen or partially frozen, warm it at room temperature until it flows normally.
- Hold the powder syringe upright and tap the barrel of the syringe to dislodge the packed powder.
- Remove the cap from the liquid syringe, then remove the cap from the powder syringe.
- Place the liquid syringe on top of the powder syringe and connect the syringes by twisting approximately ¾ turn. Keep your fingers off the plungers during this step to avoid spillage of the medication.
- Push vigorously to transfer the contents of the liquid syringe into the powder syringe. Do not wait for powder wetting and quickly start mixing contents by pushing the plungers fast and alternately for 100 pushes (two pushes within 1 second, approximately 1 minute).
- Ensure medication is passing between both syringes for proper mixing. Medication is viscous. Force needs to be applied when pressing on the plunger rods (one push equals back-and-forth between both syringes).

Table 16.4 Needle size selection [1]

Injection site	Needle size
Deltoid	1 inch (21G)
Gluteus	2 inches (20G)

- Transfer all contents into the liquid syringe.
- Maintain slight pressure on the powder syringe plunger and pull back gently on the liquid syringe plunger while twisting the syringes apart.
- Attach the safety needle by twisting it. Table 16.4 provides details on needle size for the injection sites.
- Check that the medication is uniform in color and free from foreign particles.
- Injections must be given within 15 minutes after reconstitution.
- Choose the needle and injection site.
- Clean the skin with an alcohol pad.
- Hold the syringe upright for several seconds to allow air bubbles to rise. Remove the needle sheath and slowly depress the plunger to push out the excess air from the syringe.
- Inject the medication into the deltoid or gluteal muscle. Wait a few seconds before removing the needle.
- Dispose of the syringe in an appropriate sharps container.

References

1. Risvan® [package insert]. Madrid: Laboratorios Farmaceuticos Rovi; 2024.
2. Schoretsanitis G, Bauman P, Conca A, et al. Therapeutic drug monitoring of long-acting injectable antipsychotic drugs. Ther Drug Monit. 2021;43:79–102.

Chapter 17
Olanzapine Pamoate (Zyprexa® Relprevv™): Second-Generation Antipsychotic Long-Acting Injectable

LAI Technology

Zyprexa® Relprevv™ is a crystalline salt form of olanzapine combined with pamoic acid. This crystalline salt is insoluble in water but has very low solubility in muscle tissue. When injected deeply into the gluteal muscle, the salt forms a depot at the injection site. The salt dissolves slowly at the injection site, leading to a gradual and sustained release of olanzapine into the bloodstream. Pamoic acid facilitates extended delivery but has no known pharmacological activity and is excreted unchanged [1].

Zyprexa® Relprevv™ is a long-acting atypical antipsychotic for intramuscular injection indicated for the treatment of schizophrenia [1].

Dosing Parameters

As with all long-acting injectables (LAIs), establishment of tolerability with prior oral administration is recommended prior to utilization of the LAI formulation. Table 17.1 provides dosing recommendations for Zyprexa® Relprevv™ [1].

Zyprexa® Relprevv™ has an established conversion of the oral formulation to the LAI formulation. For patients taking 10 mg of oral olanzapine daily, during the first 8 weeks, the patient would receive 210 mg every 2 weeks or 405 mg every 4 weeks. This patient would receive a maintenance dose, after the first 8 weeks of 150 mg every 2 weeks or 300 mg every 4 weeks. For patients taking 15 mg of oral olanzapine daily, during the first 8 weeks, the patient receives 300 mg every 2 weeks. This patient would receive a maintenance dose, after the first 8 weeks of 210 mg every 2 weeks or 405 mg every 4 weeks. Finally, for patients taking 20 mg orally of olanzapine daily, during the first 8 weeks, the patient would receive 300 mg every

M. J. Ehret, *Long-Acting Injectable Medications in Mental Health*,
https://doi.org/10.1007/978-3-032-09415-5_17

Table 17.1 Dosing recommendations [1]

Initial dose	Based on oral olanzapine dose
Oral overlap	Not required
Target dose	Based on oral olanzapine dose
Maximum dose	300 mg every 2 weeks; 405 mg every 4 weeks
Dosing interval	Every 2 or 4 weeks
Renal/hepatic dosing	Not studied

IM Intramuscular

Table 17.2 Pharmacokinetic properties [1, 3]

Half-life	30 days
TMax	7 days
Time to steady state	3 months
Therapeutic window	10–40 ng/mL

TMax Time to maximum concentration

2 weeks. The patient receives a maintenance dose after the first 8 weeks of 300 mg every 2 weeks.

If an individual missed a scheduled injection of Zyprexa® Relprevv™, an established missed dose schedule has been provided within the package insert. If the patient has not reached steady state, the loading dose based on the oral dose should be provided for the next 2 months. If the patient is at steady state, but it has been less than or equal to 2 months since the last injection, the next injection should be given as soon as possible. Finally, if the patient is at steady state and it has been greater than 2 months since the last injection, the loading dose based on the oral dose should be provided for the next 2 months [2].

Pharmacokinetic Properties

Table 17.2 provides pharmacokinetic properties [1, 3].

Drug Interactions

Use of CYP1A2 inducers can increase the clearance of olanzapine, with olanzapine requiring a dose increase. Utilization of concurrent CYP1A2 inhibitors can decrease the clearance of olanzapine [1].

Adverse Reactions

Zyprexa® Relprevv™ has a Risk Evaluation and Mitigation Strategies (REMS) program required for utilization of the medication. Due to a serious reaction following injection, postinjection delirium/sedation syndrome (PDSS), Zyprexa® Relprevv™ is required to be administered in a registered health care facility with ready access to emergency response services. PDSS is consistent with the signs and symptoms of olanzapine overdose, in particular, sedation (including coma) and/or delirium. After each injection, a health-care professional must continuously observe the patient at the health care facility for at least 3 hours for symptoms consistent with olanzapine overdose, including sedation and/or delirium. These symptoms may include confusion, disorientation, agitation, anxiety, cognitive impairment, extrapyramidal symptoms, dysarthria, ataxia, aggression, dizziness, weakness, hypertension, and convulsions. PDSS typically occurs due to administration of Zyprexa® Relprevv™ into the blood vasculature versus the gluteal muscle. Administration techniques are essential to the appropriate administration of this medication. The potential onset of PDSS is greatest within the first hour after injection. Following the 3-hour observation period, health-care professionals must confirm that the patient is alert, oriented, and free of any signs and symptoms of PDSS before going home. All patients must be accompanied to their destination upon leaving the health care facility. For the remainder of the day after each injection, patients should be advised not to drive or operate heavy machinery and should monitor for any signs of PDSS. If PDSS is suspected at any time, close medical supervision and monitoring should be instituted in a facility capable of resuscitation [1].

Zyprexa® Relprevv™ has similar adverse effects to the oral olanzapine products.

Preparation and Administration Instructions

Zyprexa® Relprevv™ is available as a single-dose kit in 210, 300, and 405 mg strengths. These syringes should be stored at room temperature. When the medication is suspended in the solution, it may be held at room temperature for 24 hours. The vial should be agitated immediately before product withdrawal. Once the suspension is withdrawn into the syringe, it should be used immediately.

Injection site: Gluteal muscle

Injection volume: The injection volume is based on the medication strength provided. For 150 mg, the injection volume is 1 mL, 210 mg is 1.4 mL, 300 mg is 2 mL, and 405 mg is 2.7 mL.

Administration instructions [1]:

- Must be administered as an intramuscular injection by a health-care professional. Do not administer by any other route.
- As a universal precaution, hands should be washed with soap and water prior to preparation and administration. Gloves should always be worn. Zyprexa® Relprevv™ can irritate the skin. Flush the hands with water if contact is made with skin.
- Determine the reconstitution volume required. It is important to note that there is more diluent in the vial than is needed to reconstitute the powder. This provides the diluent volumes to add to the vial.
  - If the dose is 150 mg, the vial strength to use is 210 mg, and the diluent to add is 1.3 mL.
  - If the dose is 210 mg, the vial strength to use is 210 mg, and the diluent to add is 1.3 mL.
  - If the dose is 300 mg, the vial strength to use is 300 mg, and the diluent to add is 1.8 mL.
  - If the dose is 405 mg, the vial strength to use is 405 mg, and the diluent to add is 2.3 mL.
- Loosen the powder by lightly tapping the vial.
- Open the prepackaged hypodermic needle-pro syringe and needle protection device.
- Withdraw the predetermined amount of diluent into the syringe.
- Inject the diluent into the powder vial.
- Withdraw air to equalize the pressure in the vial by pulling back slightly on the plunger in the syringe.
- Remove the needle from the vial, holding the vial upright to prevent any loss of the suspension.
- Engage the needle safety device.
- Create padding on a hard surface to cushion the tapping of the vial firmly and repeatedly on the surface until no powder is visible.
- Visually check the vial for clumps. Unsuspended powder will appear as yellow, dry clumps that may be clinging to the vial. Additional tapping may be required if large clumps remain.
- Shake the vial vigorously until the suspension appears smooth and is consistent in color and texture. The suspended product will appear yellow and opaque.
- If any foam forms during the shaking, let the vial stand to allow the foam to dissipate.
- If the product is not used right away, it should be reshaken vigorously to resuspend before use. It is stable at room temperature for up to 24 hours in the vial.
- Before administering the injection, verify with the patient that there will be someone to accompany the patient after the 3-hour observation period. If this is not confirmed, the injection should not be given.
- Refer to the information above for the final volume of injection to be administered.
- Attach a new safety needle to the syringe.
- Slowly withdraw the desired amount into the syringe. Some excess suspension will remain in the vial.

Table 17.3 Needle size selection [1]

Body type	Needle size[a]
Nonobese	1.5 inch (19G)
Obese	2 inches (19G)

[a]To assist in the prevention of clogging, a 19-gauge or larger needle must be used

- Engage the needle safety device and remove the needle from the syringe.
- Select the appropriate needle size. Table 17.3 provides the needle selection for the various body types.
- Attach the new safety needle.
- Select and prepare a site for injection in the gluteal area.
- After inserting the needle into the muscle, aspirate for several seconds to ensure that no blood appears. If any blood is drawn into the syringe, discard the syringe and the dose and begin with a new convenience kit. The injection should be performed with steady, continuous pressure.
- Do not massage the injection site.
- Dispose of the syringe in an appropriate sharps container.

References

1. Zyprexa® Relprevv™ [package insert]. Indianapolis: Eli Lilly and Company; 2023.
2. Carpenter J, Wong KK. Use a stepwise approach based on the unique properties of the specific medication. Curr Psychiatr Ther. 2018;17:11–20.
3. Schoretsanitis G, Bauman P, Conca A, et al. Therapeutic drug monitoring of long-acting injectable antipsychotic drugs. Ther Drug Monit. 2021;43:79–102.

Chapter 18
Introduction to the Use of Long-Acting Injectables in the Treatment of Substance Use Disorders

Medications for opioid use disorder (MOUD) and alcohol use disorder (AUD) are effective, but underutilized resources [1]. One option for MOUD is buprenorphine long-acting injectable (LAI), which was approved by the Food and Drug Administration (FDA) in 2017. It is given as a weekly or monthly injection and preferred by some patients and providers due to the lack of daily pill burden. Unfortunately, like other MOUD, buprenorphine LAI faces restrictions from the Drug Enforcement Administration (DEA) and maintains a Risk Evaluation and Mitigation Strategy (REMS), which may limit its use [2].

A recent survey concluded that only one-third of substance use treatment facilities offer buprenorphine LAI. Reasons given for the lack of administration include the need to administer buprenorphine within 14 days of receipt, preventing maintenance of onsite stocks and necessitating staff to manage stock, storage specifications, registration in REMS, and prior authorizations [2, 3].

Guidelines for Opioid Use Disorder

Current guidelines for the treatment of opioid use disorder (OUD) state that all FDA-approved medications for the treatment of OUD should be available to all patients. Clinicians should consider the patient's preferences, past treatment history, current state of illness, and treatment setting when deciding between the use of methadone, buprenorphine, and naltrexone. It is noted that oral naltrexone may be adversely affected by poor medication adherence and should not be used except in limited circumstances. The recommended further states that the extended-release injectable naltrexone reduces, but does not eliminate, issues with medication adherence. Providers are reminded to use new formulations as indicated and be mindful of emerging evidence as it becomes available [4].

M. J. Ehret, *Long-Acting Injectable Medications in Mental Health*,
https://doi.org/10.1007/978-3-032-09415-5_18

The Veterans Affairs/Department of Defense (VA/DOD) substance use disorder (SUD) treatment guidelines further describe that extended-release injectable buprenorphine has not been as extensively studied as the buccal and sublingual formulations, but trials have shown some improvement over placebo and comparative effectiveness to other buprenorphine formulations [5–7]. These guidelines state that there is insufficient evidence to recommend any one of the different FDA-approved formulations or routes of delivery of buprenorphine over another [7].

Guidelines for Alcohol Use Disorder

Current treatment guidelines for AUD recommend offering naltrexone (oral or extended release) or topiramate. It notes that there are two formulations of naltrexone that have not been directly compared to evaluate whether the long-acting formulation improves clinical outcomes for patients [8]. The injectable should be considered when medication adherence is a significant concern, and the patient is agreeable to receive monthly injections from the provider.

Advantages/Disadvantages of Long-Acting Injectable Formulations

While there is established efficacy for the use of both naltrexone and buprenorphine for the treatment of SUD, similar concerns exist for these formulations as do the LAI antipsychotic medications. Patient concerns, including injection site reactions, procedural discomfort, and the inconvenience of frequent clinic visits, have been documented [9]. Additionally, stigma around injections and potential limited support between injections can deter patients and providers from utilizing the formulation [10, 11]. Other limitations include systematic barriers within the health care system and regulatory and cost considerations [12, 13].

Conclusion

SUD presents a persistent public health challenge, and LAIs have the potential to transform treatment approaches. Similar to the use of LAIs in managing psychotic disorders, this formulation has the potential to offer an alternative to daily medication, support consistent treatment engagement, and provide long-term recovery. As these formulations continue to advance, health-care providers should routinely present LAIs as a viable option to all appropriate candidates, ensuring patients are informed of all available pathways to recovery.

References

1. Jones CM, Han B, Baldwin GT, et al. Use of medication for opioid use disorder among adults with past-year opioid use disorder in the US, 2021. JAMA Netw Open. 2023;6:e2327488.
2. Vidyasagar N, Bunting SR, Arora VM. Availability of long-acting injectable buprenorphine at substance use treatment facilities in 2021. JAMA. 2024;331:524–6.
3. Andraka-Christou B, Simon KI, Bradford WD, et al. Buprenorphine treatment for opioid use disorder: comparison of insurance restrictions, 2017–21: study examines insurance restrictions on buprenorphine treatment for opioid use disorder. Health Aff (Millwood). 2023;42:658–64.
4. American Society of Addiction Medicine. The ASAM national practice guideline for the treatment of opioid use disorder: 2020 focused update. J Addict Med. 2020;14(2S Suppl1):1–91.
5. Jones DE, Amick HR, Feltner C, et al. Pharmacotherapy for adults with alcohol use disorders in outpatients settings: a systematic review and meta-analysis. JAMA. 2014;311:1889–900.
6. VA/DOD Clinical Practice Guideline. Clinical practice guideline for the management of substance use disorders. Washington, DC: US. Government Printing Office; 2021.
7. Lofwall MR, Walsh SL, Nunes EV, et al. Weekly and monthly subcutaneous buprenorphine depot formulations vs daily sublingual buprenorphine with naloxone for treatment of opioid use disorder: a randomized clinical trial. JAMA Intern Med. 2018;178:764–73.
8. Haight BR, Learned SM, Laffont CM, et al. Efficacy and safety of a monthly buprenorphine depot injection for opioid use disorder: a multicentre, randomised, double-blind, placebo-controlled, phase 3 trial. The Lancet. 2019;393:778–90.
9. Johnson B, Flensburg OL, Capusan AJ. Patient perspectives on depot buprenorphine treatment for opioid addiction – a qualitative interview study. Substa Abuse Treat Prev Policy. 2022;17:40.
10. Grover S, Sahoo S, Subodh B, et al. Attitude and perceptions of patients towards long acting depot injections (LAIs). Asian J Psychiatr. 2019;44:200–8.
11. Langdon KJ, Hitch AE, Collins AB, et al. Integrating long-acting injectable treatment to improve medication adherence among persons living with HIV and opioid use disorder: study protocol. Addict Sci Clin Pract. 2023;18:60.
12. Fleddermann K, Molfenter T, Jacobson N, et al. Clinician perspectives on barriers and facilitators to implementing e-health technology in substance use disorder (SUD) treatment facilities. Subst Abuse. 2021;15:11782218211053360.
13. Flam-Ross JM, Marsh E, Weitz M, et al. Economic evaluation of extended-release buprenorphine for persons with opioid use disorder. JAMA Netw Open. 2023;6:e2329583.

Chapter 19
Naltrexone (Vivitrol®)

LAI Technology

Vivitrol® utilizes an extended-release microsphere, poly (lactic-co-glycolic acid), to deliver naltrexone, an opioid receptor antagonist, over 1 month. Medisorb, the technology utilized, allows for a slow and consistent release of medication into the bloodstream. The microspheres are injected intramuscularly via a gluteal injection and gradually break down, releasing the naltrexone [1].

Vivitrol® is indicated for the treatment of alcohol dependence in patients who are able to abstain from alcohol in an outpatient setting before initiation of treatment with Vivitrol® administration, for the prevention of relapse to opioid dependence, following opioid detoxification, and should be part of a comprehensive management program that includes psychosocial support [1].

Dosing Parameters

Before initiating Vivitrol®, a patient should be opioid-free for a minimum of 7–10 days to avoid precipitation of opioid withdrawal, which may be severe enough to require hospitalization. Patients should have access to naloxone for the emergency treatment of opioid overdose. This should be discussed with the patient and caregiver at the initial injection and at each subsequent injection [1].

There are no studies available to address switching from oral naltrexone, buprenorphine, or methadone. Some postmarketing case reports have indicated that certain patients may experience severe manifestations of precipitated withdrawal when switched from opioid therapy to opioid antagonist therapy. This effect may last for as long as 2 weeks. Providers should be prepared to manage these types of symptoms with nonopioid medications. Table 19.1 provides the dosing recommendations for Vivitrol® [1].

If a patient misses a dose, the next injection should be given as soon as possible.

M. J. Ehret, *Long-Acting Injectable Medications in Mental Health*,
https://doi.org/10.1007/978-3-032-09415-5_19

Table 19.1 Dosing recommendations [1]

Initial dose	380 mg IM
Oral overlap	Not required
Target dose	380 mg
Maximum dose	380 mg
Dosing interval	Every 4 weeks
Renal/hepatic dosing	Caution is recommended in administering Vivitrol® to patients with moderate to severe renal impairment Vivitrol® pharmacokinetics have not been evaluated in subjects with severe hepatic impairment

IM intramuscular

Table 19.2 Pharmacokinetic properties [1]

Half-life	5–10 days
TMax	Transient initial peak approximately 2 h after injection Second peak observed approximately 2–3 days later
Time to steady state	End of the dosing interval following the first injection

TMax time to maximum concentration

Pharmacokinetic Properties

Table 19.2 provides pharmacokinetic properties [1].

Drug Interactions

Before initiating Vivitrol®, an opioid-free duration of a minimum of 7–10 days is recommended to avoid precipitation of opioid withdrawal [1].

Adverse Reactions

Adverse reactions to Vivitrol® are similar in nature to those with the oral formulation. Injection site reactions have occurred and include pain, tenderness, induration, swelling, erythema, bruising, or pruritus. In some cases, these reactions have been severe. This medication must be given via deep intramuscular gluteal injection, and inadvertent subcutaneous injection may increase the likelihood of severe injection site reactions [1].

Preparation and Administration Instructions

Vivitrol® is a single-use kit available with 380 mg strength. It must be stored in the refrigerator at 2–8 °C (36–46 °F). Vivitrol® can be stored unopened in the original packaging at room temperature, 20–to 25 °C (68–77 °F), for up to 7 days before administration [1].

Injection site: Gluteal muscle
Injection volume: 4 mL
Administration instructions: [1]

- Must be administered as an intramuscular injection by a health-care professional. Do not administer by any other route.
- As a universal precaution, hands should be washed with soap and water prior to preparation and administration. Gloves should always be worn.
- Vivitrol® must be suspended only in the diluent supplied in the kit and must be administered only with one of the administration needles supplied in the kit.
- The carton needs to be removed from the refrigerator for approximately 45 min before administration to allow the product to come to room temperature.
- Firmly tap the vial on a hard surface, ensuring the powder moves freely.
- Remove the flip-caps from both vials and wipe with an alcohol swab.
- Place the 1-inch preparation needle on the syringe and withdraw 3.4 mL of the diluent from the diluent vial. Some diluent will remain in the vial.
- Inject 3.4 mL of diluent into the Vivitrol® microsphere vial.
- Mix the powder and diluent by vigorously shaking the vial for approximately 1 minute. A properly mixed suspension will be milky white, will not contain clumps, and will move freely down the walls of the vial.
- Immediately after suspension, withdraw 4.2 mL of the suspension into the syringe using the same preparation needle.
- Select the appropriate needle for a deep intramuscular injection. Table 19.3 provides the needle size for the various body types.

Table 19.3 Needle size selection [1]

Injection site	Needle size
Gluteal	Nonobese: 1.5 inch (20G) Obese: 2 inches (20G)

- Remove the preparation needle and replace it with the appropriately selected administration needle for immediate use.
- Peel the blister pouch of the selected administration needle open halfway. Grip the base of the needle, not the safety sheath. Attach the luer connection to the syringe with an easy clockwise twisting motion
- Seat the needle firmly on the needle protection device with a push and clockwise twist.
- Move the safety sheath away from the needle and toward the syringe barrel. Pull the sheath away from the needle. Do not twist the sheath. It could result in loosening the needle.
- Before injecting, tap the syringe to release any air bubbles, then push gently on the plunger until 4 mL of the suspension remains in the syringe.
- Using a circular motion, clean the injection site with the alcohol swab.
- Aspirate for blood before injection.
- If blood appears or the needle clogs, do not inject it. Change to the spare needle and administer into an adjacent site in the same gluteal region, again aspirating for blood before injection.
- Administer the suspension by deep intramuscular injection into the gluteal muscle, alternating buttocks per monthly injection.
- Dispose of the syringe in an appropriate sharps container.

Reference

1. Vivitrol® [package insert]. Waltham: Alkermes, Inc.; 2024.

Chapter 20
Buprenorphine Extended Release (Sublocade®): C-III Controlled Medication

LAI Technology

Sublocade® utilizes the Atrigel® system technology. This consists of biodegradable polymers dissolved in a liquid. After injection, it solidifies upon contact with aqueous body fluids to form a solid implant. The implant then delivers buprenorphine in a controlled fashion over an extended period of time. It is essential that this injection is not administered via vein or muscle. It must be given via a subcutaneous injection [1].

Sublocade® is indicated for the treatment of moderate to severe opioid use disorder in patients who have initiated treatment with a single dose of a transmucosal buprenorphine product or who are already being treated with buprenorphine and should be used as part of a complete treatment program that includes counseling and psychosocial support [1].

Dosing Parameters

Patients should have access to naloxone for the emergency treatment of opioid overdose. This should be discussed with the patient and caregiver at the initial injection and at each subsequent injection [1].

There are two pathways to receiving Sublocade®: induction in those not already receiving buprenorphine and transitioning from transmucosal buprenorphine [1].

M. J. Ehret, *Long-Acting Injectable Medications in Mental Health*,
https://doi.org/10.1007/978-3-032-09415-5_20

Induction in Patients Not Already Receiving Buprenorphine [1]

1. Treatment should be initiated when objective and clear signs of opioid withdrawal are evident to minimize the risk of precipitating withdrawal.
2. Patients should receive an initial dose (e.g., 4 mg) of transmucosal buprenorphine; observer for 1 hour to confirm tolerability.
3. The first injection of Sublocade® is recommended at 300 mg.
4. Monitor patients in a health care setting to assess for symptoms of worsening withdrawal and sedation.
5. On induction day, up to an additional 8 mg of transmucosal buprenorphine could be administered to manage withdrawal symptoms
6. The recommended second injection is 300 mg. The second injection may be administered as early as 1 week and up to 1 month after the initial injection.

Transition of Patients Already Receiving Transmucosal Buprenorphine [1]

1. Patients who have been on 8–24 mg daily of transmucosal buprenorphine may be transitioned to 300 mg of Sublocade®.
2. The recommended second injection dose is 300 mg. The second injection may be administered as early as 1 week and up to 1 month after the initial injection.
3. Patients established on long-term treatment and whose symptoms are controlled with 8–18 mg daily of transmucosal buprenorphine may receive 100 mg of Sublocade® as their second dose if symptoms remain controlled following the initial dose of 300 mg.

Maintenance Dose [1]

After the first two injections, the recommended maintenance dose is 100 mg monthly. A monthly maintenance dose of 300 mg may be considered in patients who tolerate 100 mg of Sublocade® monthly but do not demonstrate a satisfactory clinical response. Maintenance doses should be administered at least 26 days between injections. Table 20.1 provides details on the dosing recommendations for Sublocade®.

A patient who misses a maintenance dose should receive the next dose as soon as possible, with the following dose given at least 26 days later. Occasional delays in dosing up to 2 weeks are not expected to have a clinically significant impact on treatment effect [1].

Table 20.1 Dosing recommendations [1]

Dosing interval	Every 4 weeks
Renal/hepatic dosing	No renal dosing noted in package insert Patients with preexisting moderate to severe hepatic impairment are not candidates for treatment Patients who develop moderate to severe hepatic impairment while being treated should be monitored for several months for signs/symptoms of toxicity or overdose

Table 20.2 Pharmacokinetic properties [1]

Half-life	43–60 days
TMax	24 h after injection
Time to steady state	4–6 months

TMax time to maximum concentration

For patients in established treatment with 100 mg monthly, there may be times when a 2-month dosing interval is appropriate (e.g., extended travel); in those instances, a single 300 mg dose may be given to cover a 2-month period. Thereafter, the 100 mg monthly regimen will resume. Patients should be educated that the peak plasma level after the 300 mg dose will be higher than the usual monthly dose, and they may experience sedation or other adverse effects [1].

Pharmacokinetic Properties

After steady-state has been achieved, patients discontinuing Sublocade® may have detectable plasma and urine levels of buprenorphine for 12 months or longer. Table 20.2 provides pharmacokinetic properties [1].

Drug Interactions

Patients receiving Sublocade® should be monitored when starting or stopping any medications with CYP3A4 inhibition or induction for potential overdosing or underdosing. If concomitant use with serotonergic medications is warranted, the patient should be monitored for serotonin syndrome, particularly during treatment initiation and during dose adjustments of the serotonergic medications [1].

Adverse Reactions

The adverse effects of Sublocade® are similar in nature to those of oral buprenorphine. Additionally, Sublocade® is available only through a restricted Risk Evaluation and Mitigation Strategies (REMS) program. This is required due to the risk of serious harm or death that could result from intravenous self-administration. All health care settings and pharmacies that order and dispense Sublocade® must be certified in the REMS program. These settings and pharmacies must establish processes and procedures to verify that Sublocade® is provided directly to a health-care provider for administration by a health-care provider, and the medication is not dispensed to the patient [1].

The formulation does have injection site reactions, which are mostly manifested by pain, erythema, and pruritus. In some postmarketing case reports, injection site reactions have involved abscess, ulceration, and necrosis. The likelihood of serious injection site reactions may be increased with inadvertent intramuscular or intradermal administration [1].

Preparation and Administration Instructions

Sublocade® is available as a prefilled syringe in 100 and 300 mg strengths. Sublocade® must be stored in the refrigerator at 2–8 °C (36–46 °F). Once outside the refrigerator, it may be stored in its original packaging at room temperature for up to 12 weeks before administration. Discard if left at room temperature for longer than 12 weeks. Table 20.3 provides the injection volumes for the various strengths [1].

Injection site: Subcutaneous tissue of abdomen, thigh, buttock, or back of the upper arm

Administration instructions: [1]

- Must be administered as a subcutaneous injection by a health-care professional. Do not administer by any other route.
- As a universal precaution, hands should be washed with soap and water prior to preparation and administration. Gloves should always be worn.
- Remove from refrigerator before administration for approximately 15 minutes to reach room temperature. Do not open the foil pouch until the patient has arrived for the injection.
- Remove the foil pouch and safety needle from the carton. Open the pouch and remove the syringe.
- Check that the medication does not contain any contaminants or particles. It should be colorless to yellow or amber.
- Remove the cap from the syringe and the safety needle.
- Gently twist the needle clockwise until it is tight and firmly attached.

Table 20.3 Injection volume [1]

Medication strength	Injection volume
100 mg	0.5 mL
300 mg	1.5 mL

- Choose a body region for the injection. Ensure that the selected injection site has adequate subcutaneous tissue that is free of skin conditions.
- Clean the injection site with an alcohol swab.
- Hold the syringe upright for several seconds to allow air bubbles to rise. Due to the viscous nature of the medication, bubbles will not rise as quickly as those in an aqueous solution.
- Remove the needle cover and slowly depress the plunger to push out the excess air from the syringe. Small bubbles may remain in the medication.
- Pinch the skin around the injection area. Lift the adipose tissue from the underlying muscle to prevent accidental intramuscular injection.
- Insert the needle fully into the subcutaneous tissue. The actual angle of injection will depend on the amount of subcutaneous tissue.
- Use a slow, steady push to inject the medication. Continue pushing until all of the medication is given.
- Withdraw the needle at the same angle used for insertion and release the pinched skin.
- Do not rub the injection area after the injection.
- Instruct the patient that they may have a lump for several weeks that will decrease in size over time. Instruct the patient not to rub or massage the injection site and to be aware of the placement of any restrictive clothing.
- Dispose of the syringe in an appropriate sharps container.

Reference

1. Sublocade® [package insert]. Albany: Indivior UK Limited; 2025.

Chapter 21
Buprenorphine Extended Release (Brixadi®): C-III Controlled Medication

LAI Technology

Brixadi® uses the FluidCrystal® depot technology, which is a lipid-based formulation that forms a biodegradable liquid crystalline gel upon injection. This allows the technology to release buprenorphine at a steady rate over a 1-week or 1-month interval [1].

Brixadi® is indicated for the treatment of moderate to severe opioid use disorder in patients who have initiated treatment with a single dose of a transmucosal buprenorphine product or who are already being treated with buprenorphine and should be used as part of a complete treatment plan that includes counseling and psychosocial support [2].

Dosing Parameters

Patients should have access to naloxone for the emergency treatment of opioid overdose. This should be discussed with the patient and caregiver at the initial injection and at each subsequent injection [2].

There are two pathways to receiving Brixadi®: induction in those not already receiving buprenorphine and transitioning from transmucosal buprenorphine [2].

M. J. Ehret, *Long-Acting Injectable Medications in Mental Health*,
https://doi.org/10.1007/978-3-032-09415-5_21

Patients Not Currently Receiving Buprenorphine Treatment [2]

Recommended weekly dose is 24 mg of Brixadi® (weekly), titrated up over the first week of treatment as follows:

1. Administer a test dose of transmucosal buprenorphine 4 mg when objective signs of mild to moderate withdrawal appear.
2. If the dose is tolerated without precipitated withdrawal, administer the first dose of Brixadi® (weekly), 16 mg.
3. Administer an additional dose of 8 mg Brixadi® (weekly) within 3 days of the first dose to achieve the recommended 24 mg Brixadi® (weekly) dose.

If needed, during the first week of treatment, administer an additional 8 mg dose of Brixadi® (weekly), waiting at least 24 h after the previous injection, for a total weekly dose of 32 mg Briaxdi® (weekly).

Administer subsequent Briaxdi® (weekly) injections based on the total weekly dose that was established during Week 1. Dosage adjustments can be made at weekly appointments, with the maximum Brixadi® (weekly) dose being 32 mg.

A patient who missed a dose of Brixadi® (weekly) should receive the next dose as soon as possible. Brixadi® (weekly) should be administered at 7-day intervals.

Patients Switching from Transmucosal Buprenorphine-Containing Products to Brixadi® [2]

See table below for corresponding dose of Brixadi® when switching a patient from transmucosal buprenorphine to Brixadi® (weekly) or Brixadi® (monthly), expressing the transmucosal dose equivalents in terms of Subutex® or Suboxone® doses. Table 21.1 provides details on the dosing conversion of daily sublingual buprenorphine to Brixadi®.

Table 21.1 Dosing conversion of daily sublingual buprenorphine to Brixadi® [2]

Daily dose of sublingual buprenorphine	Brixadi® (weekly)	Brixadi® (monthly)
≤6 mg	8 mg	–
8–10 mg	16 mg	64 mg
12–16 mg	24 mg	96 mg
18–24 mg	32 mg	128 mg

Table 21.2 Dosing conversion of Brixadi® (weekly) to Brixadi® (monthly) [2]

Brixadi® (weekly)	Brixadi® (monthly)
16 mg	64 mg
24 mg	96 mg
32 mg	128 mg

Table 21.3 Dosing recommendations [2]

Dosing interval	Every week or every 4 weeks
Renal/hepatic dosing	No renal dosing noted in package insert Patients with preexisting moderate to severe hepatic impairment are not candidates for treatment Patients who develop moderate to severe hepatic impairment while being treated should be monitored for several months for signs/symptoms of toxicity or overdose

Patients Transitioning Between Brixadi® (Weekly) to Brixadi® (Monthly) [2]

See table below for the corresponding dose of Brixadi® (weekly) when converting to Brixadi® (monthly) or vice versa. Table 21.2 provides details on the dosing conversion of Brixadi® (weekly) to Brixadi® (monthly).

A patient who misses a dose of Brixadi® should receive the next dose as soon as possible. Brixadi® (weekly) should be administered in 7-day intervals. Brixadi® (monthly) should be administered in 28-day intervals. Table 21.3 provides the dosing recommendations for Brixadi®.

Pharmacokinetic Properties

Table 21.4 provides pharmacokinetic properties [2].

Table 21.4 Pharmacokinetic properties [2]

Half-life	3–5 days for weekly injection 19–26 days for monthly injection
TMax	24 h for weekly injection; 6–10 h for monthly injection

TMax time to maximum concentration

Drug Interactions

Patients receiving Brixadi® should be monitored when starting or stopping any medications with CYP3A4 inhibition or induction for potential overdosing or underdosing. If concomitant use with serotonergic medications is warranted, the patient should be monitored for serotonin syndrome, particularly during treatment initiation and during dose adjustments of the serotonergic medications [2].

Adverse Reactions

The adverse effects of Brixadi® are similar in nature to those of oral buprenorphine. Additionally, Brixadi® is available only through a restricted Risk Evaluation and Mitigation Strategies (REMS) program. This is required due to the risk of serious harm or death that could result from intravenous self-administration. All health-care settings and pharmacies that order and dispense Brixadi® must be certified in the REMS program. These settings and pharmacies must establish processes and procedures to verify that Brixadi® is provided directly to a health-care provider for administration by a health-care provider, and the medication is not dispensed to the patient [2].

The formulation does have injection site reactions, which are mostly manifested by pain, erythema, and pruritus. In some postmarketing case reports, injection site reactions have involved abscess, ulceration, and necrosis. The likelihood of serious injection site reactions may be increased with inadvertent intramuscular or intradermal administration [2].

Preparation and Administration Instructions

Brixadi® is available as a prefilled syringe in 8, 16, 24, 32, 64, 96, and 128 mg strengths. Brixadi® is stored at room temperature. Table 21.5 provides the injection volume for the various strengths [2].

Injection site: Subcutaneous tissue of the abdomen, thigh, buttock, or back of the upper arm

Administration instructions: [2]

Table 21.5 Injection volume [2]

Medication strength	Injection volume
8 mg	0.16 mL
16 mg	0.32 mL
24 mg	0.48 mL
32 mg	0.64 mL
64 mg	0.18 mL
96 mg	0.27 mL
128 mg	0.36 mL

- Must be administered as a subcutaneous injection by a health-care professional. Do not administer by any other route.
- As a universal precaution, hands should be washed with soap and water prior to preparation and administration. Gloves should always be worn.
- Remove the safety syringe components from the carton. Assemble the safety syringe. While holding the syringe guard body, insert the plunger into the body of the syringe and rotate clockwise until it is attached to the stopper inside the syringe.
- Inspect the safety syringe closely. The liquid should be clear and yellowish to yellow in color. A small bubble of air may be visible.
- Clean the injection area with an alcohol wipe.
- Grasp the safety syringe with the syringe. Carefully pull the needle cap straight off.
- Pinch the skin at the injection site between your thumb and index finger.
- Hold the syringe and insert the needle at an angle of approximately 90°. Fully insert the needle.
- Release the skin. Slowly press down the plunger head until it latches in the safety device.
- Keep the plunger pressed fully down while holding the safety syringe in place for an additional 2 seconds.
- Gently pull the needle out of the skin.
- Keep the plunger fully depressed while you carefully lift the needle straight out from the injection site.
- As soon as the needle is removed from the skin, slowly remove the thumb from the plunger.
- Allow the syringe guard to automatically cover the exposed needle.
- Dispose of the syringe in an appropriate sharps container.

References

1. Lofwall MR, Walsh SL, Nunes EV, et al. Weekly and monthly subcutaneous buprenorphine depot formulations vs daily sublingual buprenorphine with naloxone for treatment of opioid use disorder: a randomized clinical trial. JAMA Intern Med. 2018;178:764–73.
2. Brixadi® [package insert]. Plymouth Meeting: Braeburn Inc.; 2023.

Chapter 22
Approaching the Patient and Successful Utilization

When considering a long-acting injectable (LAI) medication for a patient, recovery-oriented and trauma-informed care language should be utilized. The Substance Abuse and Mental Health Services Administration (SAMHSA) defines recovery as a process of change through which people improve their health and wellness, live self-directed lives, and strive to reach their full potential [1].

From a recovery perspective, LAIs should not only be seen as a tool for preventing relapse but also to help patients work toward their established goals for their treatment. The pathway to recovery is different for each patient, and LAIs may or may not be part of that path. LAIs should be offered and discussed with each patient to allow them the opportunity to ask questions and engage in their own treatment planning [1].

A strong therapeutic alliance is a crucial part of the treatment process, and those with a trauma history may have difficulty establishing these relationships. Additionally, LAIs may be seen as actual or perceived coercive experiences, which may activate trauma-related symptoms. Providers should avoid stigmatizing language and highlight the need for the patient to choose their own preferred treatment and develop their own goals for treatment.

Before administering the first and subsequent injections, the following steps are recommended: [1]

1. Offer a step-by-step description of what the process entails and what the injection may feel like.
2. Allow the patient to choose the location of the injection when possible.
3. Asking the patient if they would like to have a family member or other person join them in the room for the injection for support.
4. Engaging them in discussion about anything else that can be offered to make the injection more comfortable.

When approaching a patient to discuss the option of an LAI, shared decision-making and motivational interviewing can assist in promoting effective

M. J. Ehret, *Long-Acting Injectable Medications in Mental Health*,
https://doi.org/10.1007/978-3-032-09415-5_22

communication, collaboration, choice, and empowerment. Shared decision-making approaches include exploring various treatment options such as LAIs, oral medications, and psychosocial treatments. Motivational interviewing for the clinician to provide the clear benefits of LAIs, even if the patient is not ready to try them. Providers should begin discussions regarding LAIs early to avoid them being seen as punishment. A clear, optimistic message should be provided describing the medication as a long-acting formulation and not as an injection. The following steps are recommended when presenting an LAI: [1]

1. Presenting the advantages compared to oral medications, such as fewer adverse effects, more effectiveness in reducing symptoms, decreased risk of hospitalization, and reduced number of medications taken daily
2. Discussing the frequency of injections
3. Directly recommending an LAI

Essential methods for continued success for patients also include educating staff on the potential benefits of LAIs and how to engage patients about this formulation of medication. All members of the interdisciplinary team should regularly discuss this formulation with patients in a positive manner. Peer specialists who have lived experience are an excellent resource to advocate for and support patients on their LAI journey [1].

Reference

1. Guide to Long-Acting Medications. Antipsychotic medications and medication-assisted treatment medications for clinicians and organizations. National Council for Mental Wellbeing; 2025.

Chapter 23
Use of Long-Acting Injectable Antipsychotics in Special Populations

Pediatric Patients

Currently, there are no long-acting injectables (LAIs) that are indicated for the pediatric population. Additionally, there are no studies in those 12 years and younger. The American Psychiatric Association's Clinical Manual of Child and Adolescent Psychopharmacology acknowledges the potential benefit of LAIs in this population who are nonadherent to oral medications but does not offer any guidance for use [1]. The American Academy of Child and Adolescent Psychiatry does cautiously recommend LAIs as a treatment option in this population with schizophrenia who have both chronic psychotic symptoms and nonadherence to oral medications [2]. A systematic review identified seven single case reports, four retrospective chart reviews, a 24-week open-label trial, and one observation prospective study which utilized LAIs in children and adolescents [3]. One hundred nineteen adolescents, aged 12–17, were treated with either a first-generation (N = 21) or second-generation (N = 53) antipsychotic injections. Nonadherence was the main rationale for starting the LAI, while lack of insight into illness was a frequent characteristic. Lack of insight is typically identified in those with early-onset illness, and it has been associated with more severe symptoms [4, 5]. The risk is high for discontinuing treatment and poor outcomes in patients [6–8]. In all the studies, LAIs were associated with improvement in the patient's symptoms.

Expert recommendations for the use of LAIs in pediatric populations are detailed below (Table 23.1).

M. J. Ehret, *Long-Acting Injectable Medications in Mental Health*, https://doi.org/10.1007/978-3-032-09415-5_23

Table 23.1 Recommendations for LAI use in pediatric populations [3]

Recommendation	Level of evidence
Use of LAIs in adolescent patients who are nonadherent to oral medications	Low
LAIs should be considered if poor insight is identified	Low
LAIs should be considered to improve tolerability in those experiencing adverse effects while demonstrating improvement in symptoms and functioning	Very low
LAIs can be an option in the presence of comorbid substance use	Low
LAIs may be beneficial in the recent or first episode of psychosis	Low
Switching to an LAI formulation may help improve the effectiveness of antipsychotic medications in some patients (either monotherapy or combined with an oral antipsychotic medication) in those with resistant or severe illness	Very low

LAI long-acting injectable

Older Adults

The aging process affects medication treatment for both clinical response and adverse effects. Changes in pharmacokinetics and pharmacodynamics factors contribute to age-related differences in response to medications [9]. These changes often necessitate the need to start at a lower dose and titrate a medication more slowly over the course of treatment. This is no different for the use of antipsychotic medications in this population. Additionally, coexisting medical illnesses and concomitant medications increase the risk for adverse effects and drug interactions. Some of the age-related differences to consider in response to medication include: delayed gastric emptying, reduced levels of plasma proteins (i.e., albumin), reduced circulatory volume, decreased circulatory volume, decreased synthesis and activity of hepatic microsomal enzymes, increased relative and absolute amount of adipose tissue, decreased body water, decreased renal blood flow, and impaired glomerular filtration and reduced medication clearance [10, 11].

Other changes as the patient ages include decreases in total body water and lean body mass with an increase in adipose tissue, which makes lipid-soluble medications such as antipsychotics have an increased volume of distribution and subsequently a prolonged time of activity. There are also changes in neurotransmitter receptors, including serotonin, alpha and beta noradrenergic, and dopamine [12]. Additionally, there is a decrease in the function of choline acetyltransferase and increased permeability of the blood-brain barrier. Each of these changes leads to the potential of increased exposure to medications, increasing the potential for adverse effects (Table 23.2).

Based on all these changes, the appropriate starting dose of an antipsychotic medication is approximately 25% of the usual adult dose [13]. Due to adverse effects (i.e., hypotension and sedation), antipsychotic medications can be given in

Table 23.2 Other common age-related pharmacokinetic changes [12]

Physiological characteristic	Age-related changes	Possible associated adverse effects
Absorption	↓ hydrochloric acid secretion, ↑ gastric pH ↓ gastric motility and emptying	Drug–drug interactions between medications can further slow gastric motility
Serum concentration	↓ lean muscle mass and total body water ↑ total fat content ↑ volume of distribution of medications	Prolonged elimination of lipophilic medications ↑ accumulation of medication
Renal function	↓ renal blood flow, glomerular filtration rate, creatinine production, clearance capacity due to tubular dysfunction	↓ clearance of some medications Accumulation of metabolites
Hepatic function	↓ hepatic blood flow, total hepatic mass, hepatic enzyme activity	↑ concentrations of unmetabolized medications–accumulation ↓ clearance of most psychotropics

Adapted from Ref. [12]

divided doses and titrated slowly. Treatment for 6 weeks or longer may be needed to achieve the optimum therapeutic effect. Total maintenance dose ranges from 25% to 50% of the usual adult dose.

Like the pediatric population, there is a paucity of data on the use of LAIs in older adults. There are three studies utilizing first-generation antipsychotic LAIs, including a total of 53 patients [14–16]. The data demonstrate that fluphenazine and haloperidol are effective in treating symptoms of schizophrenia, as well as behavioral and psychological signs of dementia, with minimal adverse effects. Lower doses are recommended due to a decreased tendency to cause sedation, postural hypotension, and anticholinergic effects compared to other typical antipsychotics [17, 18]. Common adverse effects experienced in the trials included: postural hypotension, excessive sedation, anticholinergic effects, and motor effects [19].

Second-generation LAI antipsychotics may be more appropriate for this population, as this population is more susceptible to extrapyramidal symptoms and tardive dyskinesia. Consideration must be given to the potential for metabolic symptoms that can be experienced in those with preexisting medical conditions. Two studies ($N = 194$) have been conducted with second-generation antipsychotic LAIs in the older population, with a focus on risperidone. Studies demonstrated an improvement in symptoms and resulted in lower hospitalizations compared to oral medications [20, 21].

Common adverse effects reported in a psychogeriatric service review of second-generation antipsychotic LAIs included anticholinergic and adrenergic symptoms,

Table 23.3 Considerations for use of an LAI in an older patient [22]

What size needle will be necessary?
What is the injection volume?
What is the person's body mass? Obese? More adipose versus muscle mass?
What is the route of administration? Does the patient have adequate mass at that site?
What is the angle of injection?
When landmarking the injection, you may need to measure fingers to make sure they span at least 5 cm
Identification of bony structures
Consideration of bunching or flattening techniques
Older adults and thin patients may only tolerate up to 2 mL in a single injection

dyslipidemia, hyperglycemia, and an increased risk of extrapyramidal symptoms and tardive dyskinesia [21] (Table 23.3).

Pregnant Individuals

Similar to pediatric and older people, there is a paucity of data available on evaluating the risks associated with beginning LAIs during pregnancy. There is no published data on how compounds utilized to formulate LAIs affect individuals who are pregnant or neonates [18]. It is unknown what the effect of the steady blood levels versus the daily fluctuations of antipsychotics could have on the neonate. It has been suggested that a more constant plasma medication level may reduce fetal exposure to the highly fluctuating plasma medication levels, which may improve adverse effects and outcomes [23].

Other considerations for the use of LAIs in individuals who are pregnant include the potential need for a temporary increase in dosage of some antipsychotics, given pregnancy-associated pharmacokinetic changes [24]. Additionally, aripiprazole may require higher doses or supplementation with oral medication due to the increased expression and activity of CYP2D6 during pregnancy [24]. Considerations should be given to LAIs with favorable metabolic profiles with the increase in weight that occurs during pregnancy.

The benefits of oral antipsychotics during pregnancy have been established, but the lack of information on specific risks of LAIs in pregnancy has hindered their routine use during pregnancy. There are no case-control studies, cohort studies, randomized controlled trials, or systematic reviews currently available for review. There are 12 case reports, with the majority in second-generation antipsychotics. Six neonates were born without noted complications. The other had noted complications, including intrauterine growth restriction, bilateral talipes equinovarus, and premature delivery [18]. It is hard to conclude with a small number of cases with

Table 23.4 Candidates for LAIs during pregnancy [38]

Women with histories of hospitalizations precipitated by medication nonadherence
Women with histories of frequent and extended psychiatric hospitalizations associated with schizophrenia, schizoaffective disorder, and bipolar disorder
Psychiatric decompensation during previous pregnancies, the immediate postpartum period, or a history of illicit substance abuse

many confounders. If extrapolating oral antipsychotic risk, there is a higher risk for gestational diabetes and C-section in those receiving antipsychotics while pregnant [25–27]. Additionally, prematurity, being born large for gestational age, congenital malformations, decreased neuromotor performance, withdrawal symptoms, and neonatal hospitalization were found [26–32]. While these risks with medications need to be monitored, the risks of discontinuing antipsychotics can precipitate relapses of the illness and increase the risk of postpartum psychosis, which has been associated with infanticide and maternal suicide [33–37] (Table 23.4).

Current safety data on antipsychotic use during lactation are limited but generally regarded as safe [39]. Consideration should be given to those at risk of preterm delivery, and LAIs should be avoided if a patient plans to strictly breastfeed, as preterm infants are at risk for elevated plasma medication concentrations due to immature hepatic and renal systems [40]. Pharmacologic properties of the antipsychotic medication and impact on prolactin also need to be considered, as antipsychotic induced mastitis has been reported in the literature [41].

When considering the use of an LAI in individuals who are pregnant or of childbearing age, it is essential to establish the capacity to engage in discussion of informed consent regarding the use of an LAI. The provider should review and document the current limitations of known safety data and the risks of psychiatric decompensation from untreated and undertreated illnesses. Discussion of how risks of continuation and discontinuation should include how these may affect both the pregnant individual and the developing fetus.

When selecting the appropriate LAI medication, previous efficacy of the oral formulation should be considered. Additionally, the patient's ability to be adherent with the needed time for oral overlap if required, potential adverse effects, and cost all need to be discussed. Close collaboration between the psychiatric and the obstetric teams is essential for successful outcomes.

First-Episode Psychosis

The first episode of psychosis is a critical time point in the natural course of the illness, as untreated psychosis may have untoward effects on neurobiological function, and the lack of early intervention is related to a higher rate of relapse [42]. Robinson et al. reported that 82% of patients with first episodes have a relapse in the first 5 years and that patients who discontinued their medication have a five-fold higher risk of relapse than those who remained on medication [43]. Early intervention can have a beneficial effect on the long-term outcomes for the patient, whereas delayed access to treatment or discontinuation of antipsychotic medications can increase the risk of relapses and worsen clinical outcomes [44, 45].

In the first 2 years of illness, experiencing psychotic symptoms is the strongest predictor of long-term symptoms and disability [46]. Additionally, patients may experience a decrease in treatment response with each subsequent exacerbation [47]. Neuropathological brain changes often progress with subsequent clinical episodes [48]. LAIs may decrease the time spent experiencing psychotic symptoms, decrease the number of psychotic episodes, and allow for identification of overt nonadherence and eliminate covert nonadherence [49].

A recent Delphi panel of 17 psychiatrists experienced in treating schizophrenia with LAIs recommended that all patients with schizophrenia should be evaluated clinically for LAI treatment. The panel determined that LAIs were appropriate even in those who have a high level of insight into their illness, have good social support, are currently adherent to medication, and have not had a relapse. The group concluded that the potential value of LAIs in the treatment of the first episode included decreasing the risk of relapse, rehospitalization, and functional dysfunction [50].

References

1. McVoy M, Findling RL. Clinical manual of child and adolescent psychopharmacology. Washington, DC: Amer Psychiatric Pub; 2017.
2. McClellan J, Stock S. American Academy of Child and Adolescent Psychiatry (AACAP) Committee on Quality Issues (CQI). Practice parameter for the assessment and treatment of children and adolescents with schizophrenia. J Am Acad Child Adolesc Psychiatry. 2013;52:976–90.
3. Baeza I, Fortea A, Ilzarbe D, et al. What role for long-acting injectable antipsychotics in managing schizophrenia spectrum disorders in children and adolescents? Pediatric Drugs: A systematic review; 2023.
4. Parellada M, Fraguas D, Bombin I, et al. Insight correlates in child-and adolescent-onset first episodes of psychosis: results from CAREPS study. Psychol Med. 2009;39:1433–145.
5. Parellada M, Boada L, Fraguas D, et al. Trait and state attributes of insight in first episodes of early-onset schizophrenia and other psychoses: a 2-year longitudinal study. Schizophre Bull. 2011;37:38–51.
6. Modesitt T, Kubascik E, Ott C. Extent of use of long-acting injectable antipsychotics in children and adolescents with Indiana Medicaid. Ment Health Clin. 2018;8:202–7.
7. Lincoln TM, Lullmann E, Rief W. Correlates and long-term consequences of poor insight in patients with schizophrenia. A systematic review. Schizophr Bull. 2007;33:1324–42.
8. Osatuke K, Ciesla J, Kasckow JW, et al. Insight in schizophrenia: a review of etiological models and supporting research. Compre Psychiatry. 2008;49:70–7.
9. Caligiuri MP, Jeste DV, Lacro JP. Antipsychotic-induced movement disorders in the elderly: epidemiology and treatment recommendations. Drugs Aging. 2000;17:363–84.
10. Sajatovic M, Madhusoodanan S, Buckley P. Schizophrenia in the elderly. CNS Drugs. 2000;13:103–15.

11. Drenth-van Maanen A, Wilting I, Jansen PAF. Prescribing medicines to older people-how to consider the impact of ageing on human organ and body functions. Br J Clin Pharmacol. 2020;86:1921–30.
12. Balaram K, Balachandran S. Psychopharmacology in the elderly: why does age matter? Psychiatric Clin N Am. 2022;45:735–44.
13. Keepers GA, Fochtmann LJ, Anzia JM, et al. The American Psychiatric Association practice guideline for the treatment of patients with Schizophrenia. Am J Psychiatry. 2020;177:868–72.
14. Altamura AC, Mauri MC, Girandi T, et al. Clinical and taxological profile of fluphenazine in elderly chronic schizophrenia. Int J Clin Pharmacol Res. 1990;10:223–8.
15. Finkel SI. Antipsychotics: old and new. Clin Geriatr med. 1998;14:87–100.
16. Raskind M, Alvarez C, Herlin S. Fluphenazine enanthate in the treatment of late paraphrenia. J Am Geriatr Soc. 1979;27:459–63.
17. Tran-Johnson TK, Krull AJ, Jeste DV. Late-life schizophrenia and its treatment: pharmacologic issues in older schizophrenia patients. Clin Geriatr Med. 1992;8:401–10.
18. O'Sullivan DL, Byatt N, Dossett EC. Long-acting injectable antipsychotic medications in pregnancy: a review. J Acad Consult Liaison Psychiatry. 2022;63:53–60.
19. Doolabh U, Yeap S. Examining long-acting injectable antipsychotic (depot) medication in the elderly: a five-year retrospective cross-sectional study evaluating depot use in an Australian psychogeriatric service. Aust Psychiatry. 2022;30:31–6.
20. Lasser R, Bossie C, Gharabawi G, et al. Remission in schizophrenia: results from a 1-year study of long-acting risperidone injection. Schizphr Res. 2005;77:215–27.
21. Lin CH, Chen FC, Chan HY, et al. A comparison of long-acting injectable antipsychotics with oral antipsychotics on time to rehospitalization within 1 year of discharge in elderly patients with schizophrenia. Am J Geriatr Psychiatry. 2020;28:23–30.
22. Davidson KM, Bertram JEA. Best practice for deltoid intramuscular injections in older adults: study in cadavers. J Nurs Educ Pract. 2019;9:92.
23. Ereshefsky L, Mascarenas CA. Comparison of the effects of different routes of antipsychotic administration on pharmacokinetics and pharmacodynamics. J Clin Psychiatry. 2003;64:18–23.
24. Westin AA, Brekke M, Molden E, et al. Treatment with antipsychotics in pregnancy: changes in drug disposition. Clin Pharmacol Ther. 2018:477–84.
25. Boden R, Lundgren M, Brandt L, et al. Antipsychotics during pregnancy. Arch Gen Psychiatry. 2012;69:715–21.
26. Ellfolk M, Leinonen MK, Gissler M, et al. Second-generation antipsychotics and pregnancy complications. Eur J Clin Pharmacol. 2020;76:107–15.
27. Resi M, Kallen B. Maternal use of antipsychotics in early pregnancy and delivery outcome. J Clin Psychopharmacol. 2008;28:279–88.
28. Kulkarni J, Worsley R, Gilbert H, et al. A prospective cohort study of antipsychotic medications in pregnancy. the first 147 pregnancies and 100 one year old babies. PLoS One. 2014;9:e94788.
29. Sadowski A, Todorow M, Brojeni PY, et al. Pregnancy outcomes following maternal exposure to second-generation antipsychotics given with other psychotropic drugs: a cohort study. BMJJ Open. 2013;3:e003062.
30. Johnson KC, LaPrarie JL, Brennan PA, et al. Prenatal antipsychotics exposure and neuromotor performance during infancy. Arch Gen Psychiatry. 2012;69:784–94.
31. Wisner KL, Schaefer C. Psychotropic drugs. Drugs during pregnancy and lactation. 3rd ed. London: Academic; 2015. p. 293–339.
32. Sutter-Dallay AL, Bales M, Pambrun E, et al. Impact of prenatal exposure to psychotropic drugs on neonatal outcomes in infants of mothers with serious psychiatric illness. J Clin Psychiatry. 2015;76:967–73.
33. Gitlin M, Nuechterlein K, Subotnik KL, et al. Clinical outcome following neuroleptic discontinuation in patients with remitted recent-onset schizophrenia. Am J Psychiatry. 2001;158:1835–42.

34. Viguera AC, Whitfield T, Baldessarini RJ, et al. Risk of recurrence in women with bipolar disorder during pregnancy: prospective study of mood stabilizer discontinuation. Am J Psychiatry. 2007;164:1817–24.
35. Spinelli MG. Maternal infanticide associated with mental illness: prevention and the promise of saved lives. Am J Psychiatry. 2004;161:1548–77.
36. Jones I, Chandra PS, Dazzan P, et al. Bipolar disorder, affective psychosis, and schizophrenia in pregnancy and the post-partum period. Lancet. 2014;384:1789–99.
37. Bergink V, Rasgon N, Wisner KL. Postpartum psychosis: madness, mania, and melancholia in motherhood. Am J Psychiatry. 2016;173:1179–88.
38. Reinstein SA, Cosgrove J, Malekshahi T, et al. Long-acting injectable antipsychotic use during pregnancy: a brief review and concise guide for clinicians. J Clin Psychiatry. 2020;81:20ac13597.
39. Kronenfeld N, Berlin M, Shaniv D, et al. Use of psychotropic medications in breastfeeding women. Birth Defects Res. 2017;109:957–97.
40. Marks JM, Spatz DL. Medications and lactation: what PNPs need to know. J Pediatr Health Care. 2003;17:311–7.
41. Nikolaev A, Blake CN, Carlson DL. Association between hyperprolactinemia and granulomatous mastitis. Breast J. 2016;22:224–31.
42. Karson C, Duffy RA, Erama A, et al. Long-term outcomes of antipsychotic treatment in patients with first-episode schizophrenia: a systematic review. Neuropsychiatr Dis Treat. 2016;12:57–67.
43. Robinson DG, Woemer MG, Delman HM, et al. Pharmacological treatments for first-episode schizophrenia. Schizophre Bull. 2005;31:705–22.
44. Salgueiro M, Segarra R. Long-acting injectable second-generation antipsychotics in first-episode psychosis: a narrative review. Int Clin Psychopharmacol. 2019;34:51–6.
45. Penttila M, Jaakelainen E, Hirvonen N, et al. Duration of untreated psychosis as predictor of long-term outcome in schizophrenia: a systematic review and meta-analysis. Br J Psychiatry. 2014;205:88–94.
46. Harrison G, Hopper K, Craig T, et al. Recovery from psychotic illness: a 15-and 25-year international follow-up study. Br J Psychiatry. 2001;178:506–17.
47. Lieberman JA, Alvir JM, Koreen A, et al. Psychobiologic correlates of treatment response in schizophrenia. Neuropsychopharmacology. 1996;14:13S–21S.
48. Lieberman JA, Drake RE, Sederer LI, et al. Science and recovery in schizophrenia. Psychiatr Serv. 2008;59:487–96.
49. Fenton WS, Blyler CR, Heinssen RK. Determinants of medication compliance in schizophrenia: empirical and clinical findings. Schizophre Bull. 1997;23:637–51.
50. Arango C, Fagiolini A, Gorwood P, et al. Delphi panel to obtain clinical consensus about using long-acting injectable antipsychotics to treat first-episode and early-phase schizophrenia: treatment goals and approaches to functional recovery. BMC Psychiatry. 2023;23:453.

Chapter 24
Switching and Discontinuing Long-Acting Injectable Antipsychotics

Switching Between Long-Acting Injectables

In the perfect setting, a long-acting injectable (LAI) antipsychotic medication is initiated after an established dose was determined to be efficacious and tolerable in a patient. Many times, this is not the case, and health-care professionals are required to switch LAIs during a patient's treatment. There are several strategies to consider when determining how to design a treatment plan for switching between the various formulations. See Fig. 24.1 for an algorithm for switching between LAIs and Table 24.1 for considerations when switching between LAIs.

Specific details on how to switch between LAIs that are available in the package labeling have been detailed in the specific medication chapters. Research has demonstrated that in those patients who have achieved a steady state with a first-generation LAI, plasma concentrations will stay relatively consistent for 6–7 weeks since the previous injection, which may suggest that the next injection with the new LAI may not need to be administered until that time [1–4]. For many second-generation LAIs, the next injection should be given on the date of the next injection. There are several exceptions to this rule: risperidone microspheres, risperidone extended-release injectable suspension, and paliperidone palmitate every 3–6 months. See chapter-specific information for details. No guidance exists for aripiprazole LAI medications; however, based on the pharmacokinetic data, administration of the next LAI should be given on the date of the next injection.

In addition to the utilization of pharmacokinetic data and recommendations from the package insert, therapeutic medication levels can be instrumental in determining when to administer the next LAI [5–7]. Obtaining a therapeutic medication level on the date of the next injection can assist the clinician in determining the release of the previous medication specific to that patient. Based on the determined level and the current symptomatology, the provider could choose to provide the new injection or

M. J. Ehret, *Long-Acting Injectable Medications in Mental Health*,
https://doi.org/10.1007/978-3-032-09415-5_24

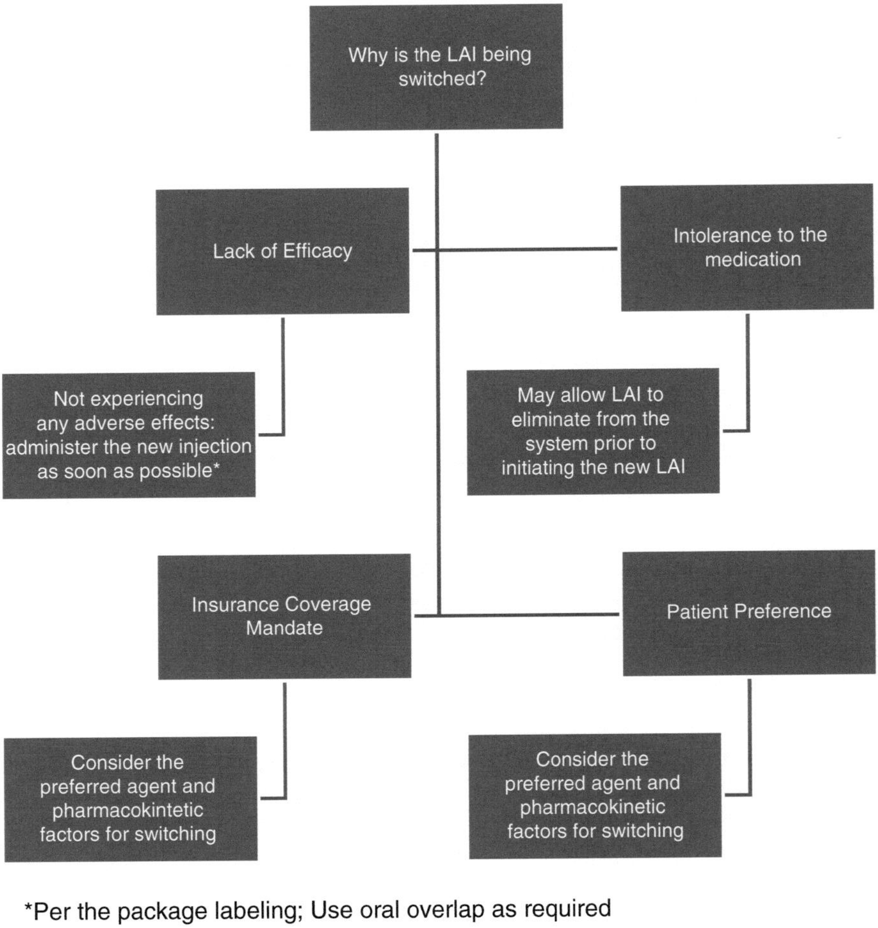

Fig. 24.1 Algorithm for switching between LAIs. *Per the package labeling: use oral overlap as required

Table 24.1 Factors for consideration when switching between LAIs

Which LAI will be selected for the next injection?
When will the next injection be administered? Is there any guidance provided in the package insert labeling?
What is the half-life and release mechanism of the current LAI the patient is receiving?
What are the oral overlap requirements, if necessary, for the new LAI?
What was the date of the last LAI injection?

wait until the plasma level drops further in the patient. See the chapter-specific medication chapters for established therapeutic levels.

Discontinuing Long-Acting Injectables

In the ideal setting, patients who are stabilized on an LAI would stay on this formulation for the duration of their treatment. Unfortunately, at times, an LAI will need to be discontinued. There is a paucity of data regarding how to discontinue an LAI. There is neither a consensus nor a recognized guideline advising how and when to discontinue an LAI and restart an oral antipsychotic.

Before discontinuing an LAI antipsychotic, the interdisciplinary team should review with the patient and caregivers the risks and benefits of switching medication formulations, including the risk of decompensation and potential adverse effects [8]. There are several established steps in the discontinuation process, starting with determining whether the patient will continue the same oral medication as the LAI antipsychotic or if a different oral antipsychotic will be initiated. The next step is to determine when to initiate the oral medication. This requires obtaining several pieces of information including the oral dose equivalent of the patient's current LAI, the half-life of the LAI, and the release mechanism of the LAI. Additionally, the date of the last injection should be obtained. All pharmacokinetic information on specific medications is available in the medication-specific chapters.

As research has shown, patients who have achieved a steady state with first-generation antipsychotics, plasma concentrations stay relatively consistent for 6–7 weeks after the last injection, and oral medications may not need to be initiated until that time [1–4]. For many second-generation antipsychotic LAIs, oral medication may be initiated on the date of the next injection. The exception would be the risperidone microspheres, which have a delayed release of either 7 or 21 days. Once a patient is at a steady state with risperidone microspheres, trough levels are not observed until 1 week or 3–4 weeks after discontinuation, depending on the product utilized [9]. Similar to switching between LAIs, utilizing therapeutic drug levels can be instrumental in determining the data regarding the release of the medication specific to the individual patient. Based on the obtained level and the current symptomatology, the health-care provider could choose to start the oral medication at a lower dose and titrate back to the LAI equivalent oral dose or initiate the oral dose at the LAI equivalent oral dose.

References

1. Gitlin MJ, Midha KK, Fogelson D, et al. Persistence of fluphenazine in plasma after decanoate withdrawal. J Clin Psychopharmacol. 1988;8:53–6.
2. Wistedt B, Jorgensen A, Wiles D. A depot neuroleptic withdrawal study. Plasma concentration of fluphenazine and flupentixol and relapse frequency. Psychopharmacology. 1982;78:301–4.
3. Chang WH, Lin SK, Juang DJ, et al. Prolonged haloperidol and reduced haloperidol plasma concentrations after decanoate withdrawal. Schizophr Res. 1993;9:35–40.
4. Eklund K, Forsman A. Minimal effective dose and relapse-double-blind trial: haloperidol decanoate vs. placebo. Clin Neuropharmacol. 1991;1:S7–S15.
5. Taylor D, Barnes TRE, Young AH. The Maudsley prescribing guidelines in psychiatry. 13th ed. Wiley-Blackwell; 2018.
6. Schoretsanitis G, Bauman P, Conca A, et al. Therapeutic drug monitoring of long-acting injectable antipsychotic drugs. Ther Drug Monit. 2021;43:79–102.
7. Meyer JM, Stahl SM. The clinical use of antipsychotic plasma levels. Cambridge University Press; 2021.
8. Ehret MJ, Carr CC. Discontinuing a long-acting injectable antipsychotic: what to consider. Curr Psychiatr Ther. 2023;22:35–8.
9. Wilson WH. A visual guide to expected blood levels of long acting injectable risperidone in clinical practice. J Psychiatr Pract. 2004;10:393–401.

Index

M. J. Ehret, *Long-Acting Injectable Medications in Mental Health*,
https://doi.org/10.1007/978-3-032-09415-5

MIX
Papier aus verantwortungsvollen Quellen
Paper from responsible sources
FSC® C105338

If you have any concerns about our products,
you can contact us on
ProductSafety@springernature.com

In case Publisher is established outside the EU,
the EU authorized representative is:
Springer Nature Customer Service Center GmbH
Europaplatz 3, 69115 Heidelberg, Germany

Printed by Libri Plureos GmbH
in Hamburg, Germany